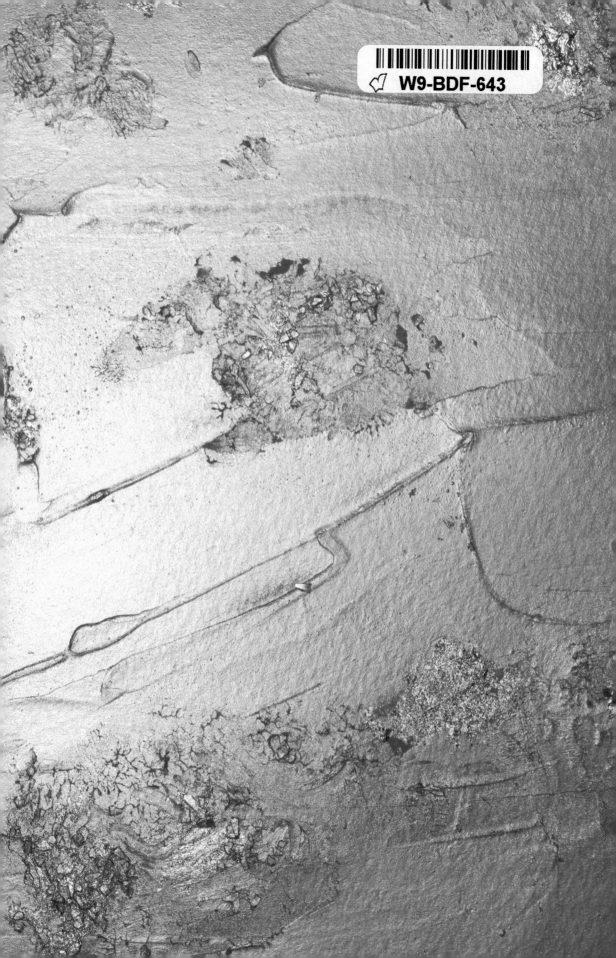

W9-BDF-643

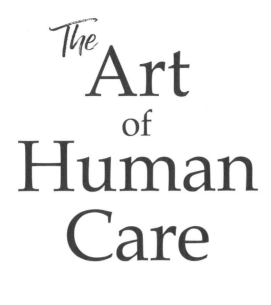

The Art of Human Care

for COVID-19

HASSAN A. TETTEH

With UNDERSTANDING SOWERBY

©Copyright 2021

All Rights Reserved.
No part of this book may be reproduced in any manner
without the author's express written consent except
in the case of brief excerpts in critical reviews and articles.

The opinions and assertions expressed herein are those of
the author(s) and do not necessarily reflect the official policy
or position of the United States Navy, Uniformed Services
University, or the Department of Defense.

Inquiries about this book should be addressed to:
TCG Publishing
Bethesda, Maryland, USA
(800) 838-7061

www.doctortetteh.com

The Art of Human Care for COVID-19
Hassan A. Tetteh
with Understanding Sowerby
ISBN: 978-1-7336654-5-2
Library of Congress Control Number: 2020920124

Written by Hassan A. Tetteh
Cover Design by Karen McDiarmid | Book Design by Karen McDiarmid
Illustrated by Understanding Sowerby & Massah Fofana

Printed in Canada

10 9 8 7 6 5 4 3 2 1

for

Carmen Santana
and
Gregory "Dad" Lewis

Ars longa, vita brevis.
—Hippocrates

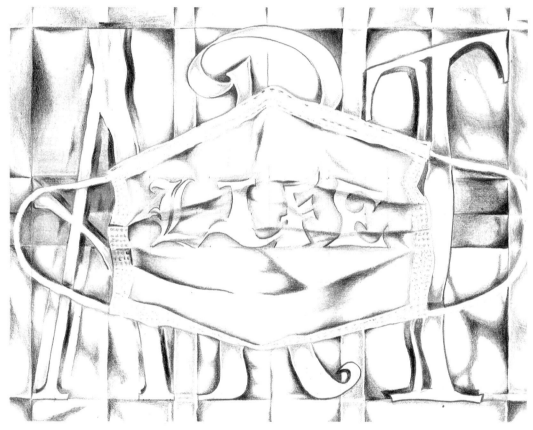

ART IS LONG: Understanding Sowerby

Translation:
Art is long, life is short.

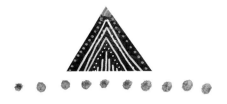

Contents

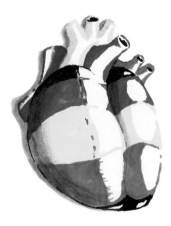

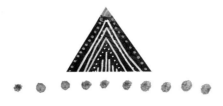

Foreword

Estelle Slootmaker

Writer, editor, and *Second Wave Michigan* journalist

In a January 2021 phone meeting to discuss this book, Dr. Tetteh shared his experience of the 9/11 attacks on New York City's Twin Towers. He was on the trauma team waiting for anticipated casualties and took a break on the roof of Kings County Hospital, looking over the city, when he saw the first World Trade Center tower collapse … and then the second. After recovering from the initial shock, his thoughts immediately raced to his sister, who worked in one of the towers. A few frantic phone calls later, he learned that, due to car trouble, she had not been able to get to work that day. Hassan pointed out to me that while more than 3,000 Americans lost their lives on that day, COVID-19 was killing well over 3,000 Americans every day during the time we were working on this book.

As I write this foreword on January 19, 2021, more than 400,000 Americans have succumbed to the virus and more than 2 million worldwide. Hassan's experience with COVID-19 has been equally personal and professional. As a physician, he served on the front lines, treating patients in the throes of the disease. As a husband

and father, he saw his wife laid off from her job and helped supervise his two children as they home-schooled. Unlike 9/11, when good fortune or some greater power kept his sister from harm, the COVID-19 pandemic has not spared his family. Hassan lost two very dear aunts and one very close uncle. And, as a citizen scientist, he has been baffled by those in his own circle who did not take the pandemic seriously.

Assailed on all fronts, as it were, if anyone were to lose hope or become a cynic, Dr. Tetteh had the right. Instead, he chose the path of hope. Sustained by his own knowledge of past pandemics and encouraged by *The Art of Human Care* theory he had developed over his career, Dr. Tetteh invites us to join him in imagining how we can come out better on the other side of these trying times. He celebrates the positive changes that are possible because of what we've learned through this ordeal. Indeed, COVID-19 has shone a bright light upon the everyday experience of racial injustice and inequitable access to nutritious food, quality education, and medical and mental healthcare. We now have opportunity to make systemic change.

Hassan also points out that COVID-19 has reminded us of what really matters in life. Now that we know, we will choose to keep our loved ones closer. In addition, COVID-19 has given rise to innovations like telehealth and outdoor dining enclosures while emphasizing the value of virtual learning and the telecommute.

Dr. Tetteh is not alone in this positive message. As a writer for the Michigan Health Endowment Fund *State of Health Series,* I have spoken with the Michiganders who are making similar strides against and in spite of COVID. The Michigan Coronavirus Task Force on Racial Disparities has dramatically reduced COVID-19 cases and deaths among people of color. Medical and mental health providers turned on the dime to provide timely, effective telemedicine consults. Food banks and emergency food pantries increased services up to 300% in some locations while farmers and farmers' markets figured out how to get healthy local produce to their neighbors in need via online platforms that they had never dealt with before. Michigan's Area Agencies on Aging have even deployed robotic pets to nursing home residents experiencing loneliness and isolation. These people and their counterparts across the United States are taking the steps that will not only help us to survive this pandemic but build a healthier, more compassionate society on the other side.

However, in Dr. Tetteh's words, "It's no walk in the park." So, I invite you to read the pages before you. This book, *The Art of Human Care for COVID-19*, leads the charge. Through his own professional and personal experience of COVID-19, Hassan has found even more solace and inspiration in the simple formula for success that he spelled out in his prior book, *The Art of Human Care*. Find your purpose. Personalize your work to yourself and those you encounter. And forge partnerships to make it happen. Whether you are a ranking physician in a large healthcare system, a teacher guiding a group of youngsters, or a nonprofit volunteer connecting people with resources, this little volume has the wisdom to guide you through the days ahead.

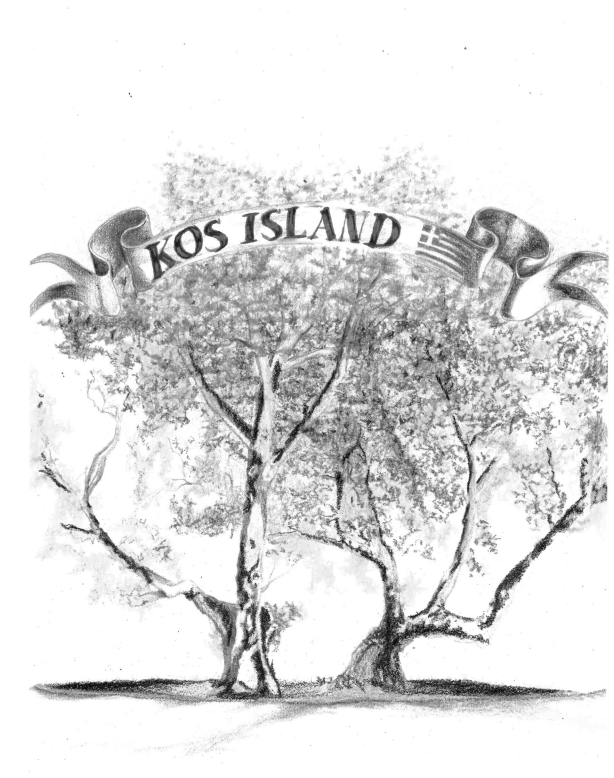

ISLAND OF KOS TREE OF HIPPOCRATES: Understanding Sowerby

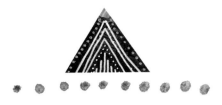

Introduction

Hassan A. Tetteh

As the present world struggles with the COVID-19 pandemic, we must not forget the past. Plagues and pandemics are nothing new. Medical advances made since the Bubonic Plague (1300s), the Spanish Flu Pandemic (1918), and even West Africa's Ebola Pandemic (2014–2016) may cause us to dismiss the methods that medical professionals of those times used to combat them. However, each of these events is quite relevant to what is happening now. Indeed, our healing professions' most ancient history continues to inform us on how to stay present with the victims of COVID-19 today.

Let me take you back to the moment in time that inspired my work. More than 2,300 years ago, the father of modern medicine, Hippocrates (459–424 BCE), received his medical training on Kos, a Greek island on the trade route between Egypt, Syria, Cyprus, and Anatolia. I visited Kos some years ago. There the Tree of Hippocrates grows, the place where he purportedly taught his students. I liberated a leaf from the tree and saved it as a reminder of what I had learned during my experience on Kos.

In my previous book, *The Art of Human Care*, I shared the story of Hippocrates' patient, Nikias, a 39-year-old businessman who felt a great pain in his chest. Nikias' father and grandfather had experienced similar chest pain before dying, both at the age of 40.

After an exhausting and ineffective in-patient visit with the healers at the Temple of Asclepius, Nikias left to go home—and collapsed at the bottom of the temple stairs. There, he met Hippocrates, who offered to help. Nikias asked him, "If you are a doctor, why aren't you practicing in the healing Temple?" Hippocrates replied, "Oh, they don't practice my kind of medicine in the Temple." Nikias returned home feeling better than he had in a long time and continued to follow Hippocrates' advice.

Hippocrates' approach was holistic in nature and built on medical knowledge he gleaned from the ancient Egyptians. He and those studying under him ushered in an era of scientific inquiry and organized knowledge as well as the art of diagnosis and healing.

Hippocrates, now known as the Father of Modern Medicine, also had experience with a pandemic. You may recall the movie, *300: Rise of an Empire,* which tells the story of how the Spartans conquered Athens during the Peloponnesian War (431–405 BCE). While the movie would have you think that superior military strategy, physical prowess, and mastery of the war technologies of the times overcame Athens, the city's medical history gives a somewhat different account.

A War Story: The Fall of Athens and COVID-19

During my master's degree studies in National Security Strategy at the National War College, my classmates lauded the generals

and brilliant military minds endowed with the strategies and technologies to win the great wars of the past. My contribution to these conversations generally centered on how viruses, disease, illness, and pandemics had played an equally important role. As you can imagine, at the War College, we studied war and national security. We went back in history to study wars like the Peloponnesian War and also discussed modern campaigns.

In every one of these campaigns, my classmates talked about the brilliance of the strategist, the tactical advantages, and the weapons. I always looked for the health angle—and how, in every case, that was the decisive factor. True, the military strategies, technology, logistics, and leadership were influential and very powerful. However, health issues, and specifically war-fighter health, also had a great impact on the outcomes of the campaigns we studied. My classmates would roll their eyes and say, "Here goes the doc talking about these pandemics and things again. We've got to listen to the doc tell us about the Peloponnesian War."

But how did that small island of Sparta defeat Athens? Think about it—a little island versus the center of Greek civilization. It was like a little Caribbean island beating the United States. I offered, "Consider the reason why Athens failed. Before those decisive battles, if you recall, Athens experienced a devastating plague."

To deal with the plague, Athens closed its walls and kept everyone inside. The disease spread like wildfire throughout the population. It took out Athens' greatest statesmen and leaders, even Pericles. Think about what a giant force he was in that civilization. He died. The plague wiped him out.

Athens was left with inexperienced leaders who were not very wise and who, due to the death and devastation they had witnessed, had lost their faith and their moral compass. So, the little Spartan island beat great Athens. Well, that's how the story goes. We will sensationalize it in movies like *300: Rise of an Empire*. We like the buff warriors and story of how they did it. However, I think the plague was very consequential and contributed to the defeat of Athens.

The Athenians' spirit was destroyed before the Spartans ever arrived. Why? Because they had lost faith in God, because they were feeling, "How could there be a god if we're all dying like this?" Think about living in a civilization and a society that has come to that kind of despair—citizens down on their knees from this death and plague. Anybody could have come in there and wiped them out.

So, what is the connection to today? The connection is that society fundamentally changes with each one of the global pandemic events. How you adapt, emerge, and how you evolve has consequences. How society collectively adapts, emerges, and evolves from a pandemic has global consequences and impacts lives for generations.

And what does the story of Nikias and Hippocrates have to do with the practice of medicine today, especially during the time of COVID-19? Everything. How can a story from 2,300 years ago relate to the events of 2020? Well, the beginnings of modern medicine more than two millennia ago changed the world. The practice of modern medicine today, with revolutionary vaccine technology, can continue to change the world—as long as we do not stray too far from the roots of that ancient tree. In the following chapters, we will reflect upon those roots of **purpose, personalization,** and **partnerships** while considering how we can do our best in the midst of today's pandemic.

To guide that reflection, I invite you to enjoy, study, and learn from the art throughout this book. If you have read *The Art of Human Care*, you know that my childhood career choice was not to be a doctor, but an artist. While the medical profession has proven to be my true calling, I also consider healing as my art. My hope is that the art shared throughout this book will express how we need to respond to and learn from this crisis in ways words alone cannot express.

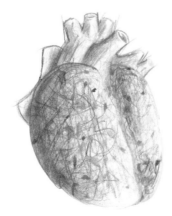

Create the Art

I wanted to be an artist when I grew up

I tagged trains in Brooklyn
And was called a hoodlum
And worked hard to show them, I could be more
I learned I could be more

I wanted to be an artist when I grew up

I almost died when I was 20, was rejected by plenty
Lost my dad and all hope in many,
Then I found an answer in the trinity-mind, body, and spirit
I learned about humility and embraced—the divinity

I wanted to be an artist when I grew up

Joined the Navy and saw combat, came back home,
but no one said that

I would be different
That things would be different
That the world would be different
I learned maybe I could be different
I learned that I could be the difference
I learned that I could make a difference
I knew I could make a difference

I wanted to be an artist when I grew up, I

Could find purpose in art
Should personalize the art
Would become a partner with art
I knew I had to start, because I
Learned I could heal with art

Life is short, but art is long

Yeah, I wanted to be an artist when I grew up,
And He gave me the power to release the bars
and the art within me
So, now I've learned I can be an artist

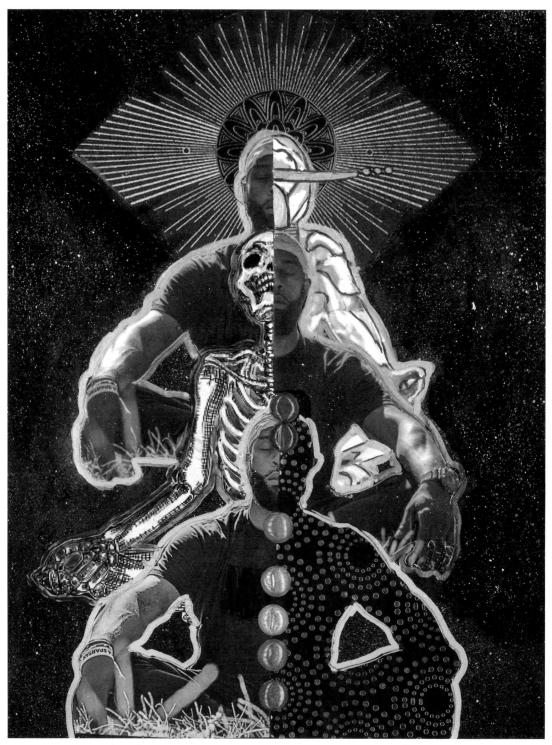

BLACK DEATH: Massah Fofana

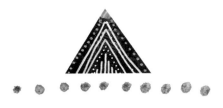

Chapter 1

Historical Perspective

The Black Death, AIDS, Ebola, and *Contagion*

As a student of pandemics, I've learned a lot from medieval and other scholars. Purdue University's Professor Dorsey Armstrong's instruction on the Black Death was incredibly informative and helpful to place COVID-19 into the appropriate context. For example, Professor Armstrong highlights what happened when the Black Death struck the medieval world in the middle of the 14th century. She notes the impact of the Black Death was on multiple levels immediate—catastrophic, and devastating. Skilled laborers and artisans died, and their knowledge was lost to the world forever.

Likewise, COVID-19 has claimed the lives of so many. We lost Charley Pride, an African American musical pioneer and the first black member of the Country Music Hall of Fame. We lost Broadway star Nick Cordero. Many followed his family's grief

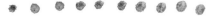

on Instagram. The lost talent of the millions of others who have died has changed the world. The medieval world coped with this unpredecented loss of skills by reinventing itself politically, economically, socially, and technologically. The social structures that had been firmly in place for centuries had become only an idea or a suggestion and no longer a reality. Individuals from the lower classes took advantage of new opportunities for upward mobility. We are seeing the same phenomenon with COVID-19 today.

Scholars like Armstrong believe the pandemic crisis ushered in the 16th-century age known as the Renaissance. Additionally, the late great historian David Hurley suggested that without the Black Death, many significant advances, including the technologies and discoveries of the European Renaissance, would have been delayed for centuries. Hurley's theory concludes the medieval world would have maintained its customs, social classes, antiquated technologies, and old political infrastructure quite easily. An outside force, like a pandemic, was necessary to change all the prior norms dramatically.

Indeed, COVID-19 has advanced many technologies, such as Zoom, Teams, and the adoption and maturation of tele-education and telemedicine.

The Black Death Plague, caused by the Yersinia pestis bacterium, changed things so rapidly in some places that its devastating impacts happened overnight. The pandemic served to fundamentally alter the social order of the past, just as COVID-19 is changing the social order of today. During the Black Death, loss of life impacted the church as well as the general population. People dissatisfied with the church before the plague became even more disappointed. Even devout followers reconsidered the meaning

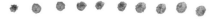

of the church's many failures during the Black Death. This kind of thinking influenced the German priest Martin Luther. Consequently, in 1517, Luther nailed his 95 Theses to the church door at Wittenberg, thus launching the Reformation and establishing Protestant denominations within Christianity, which Rome had dominated throughout its prior history.

Today, many may think the Black Death plague is gone and no longer presents a real threat to the modern world. This belief may be true. However, in the 21st century, COVID-19 demonstrates how understanding the Black Death and previous pandemics is essential today.

Contagion: The Diseases We Cannot Treat

Steven Soderbergh's 2011 *Contagion*, the American thriller film about a devastating global pandemic, had renewed popularity during COVID-19 with increased views on streaming platforms during 2020. Although *Contagion* was a fictional work, its renewed popularity highlights the art's power to both entertain and inform.

In the film, *Contagion's* cast of scientists faces the common basic human fears about disease and the terrifying possibility that we may encounter something we cannot treat. In critical moments of the film, Kate Winslet's character, Dr. Erin Mears, is the earnest and talented Epidemic Intelligence Service Officer diligently seeking the virus's etiology. She becomes both a hero and martyr, eventually losing her life to the disease. In the film, she conveys to both the people she encounters through her epidemiology work— and the audience watching—how this pandemic is different. Dr. Mears' assessment is right, but she's also wrong. Every plague, including COVID-19, almost certainly seems different from any that came before for those living through it. For them, the experience is like the end of the world.

Professor Armstrong highlights how a particularly horrible plague, the Black Death, periodically appeared and disappeared over three centuries. She outlines how no one knew when an outbreak was truly over. After 300 years of this uncertainty, no one individual dared to hope that the current outbreak might be the last. So, when the plague finally ended in London in 1666, no one celebrated. No one expressed relief. The people continued to wait for what was coming next. For the foreseeable future, many impacted by COVID-19 today will be waiting for what might come next.

When those who had survived the Black Death began to believe the plague was over for their world, other diseases filled that vacuum. For example, smallpox cases were recorded as early as 1000 BCE. However, smallpox didn't make a severe incursion into western Europe until the 16th century—during a time when the plague still recurred periodically with diminished virulence. Simultaneously, during the 16th century, two other diseases, syphilis and cholera, impacted the European population. By the end of the 19th century, Armstrong recounts how the Black Plague resurfaced in India and China without too much consequence and provided scientists with insight into the its causative agent, Yersinia pestis.

In the next century, the worldwide influenza outbreak of 1918 came on the scene, and an estimated 3–5% of planet earth's total population died before the pandemic came to an end. John Barry comprehensively recounts the story of one of history's deadliest pandemics in his acclaimed work, *The Great Influenza*. While later outbreaks of influenza, many of them severe, continued to occur, none has reached the 1918 pandemic level—yet.

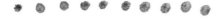

How the Black Plague Informed the HIV/AIDS Epidemic

By the end of the 20th century, lessons learned from the Black Plague, began to be promulgated. For example, the practice of quarantine came into existence with the medieval Black Death. The past plagues give people a language to talk about new diseases like HIV/AIDS and COVID-19. A review of articles written in the 1980s and 1990s by medieval literary scholars and modern social historians illustrate how Black Death and HIV frequently are mentioned together. When scholars attempted to convey the horrors of the Black Plague to their audiences, they used the example of HIV/AIDS to give a commensurate access point to the conversation and a way to relate. Armstrong, modern social historians, and others who sought to explain the consequence of HIV/AIDS in the context of contemporary psychosocial relations used the Black Death's medieval response as a kind of framework.

As that framework required some revision to be applied to HIV/AIDS, the same modifications can help us conceptualize the modern-day reactions to COVID-19. The Black Death plague in medieval Europe is a useful guide for those working on modern epidemics, like HIV/AIDS, and certainly pandemics like COVID-19 that are still in progress.

Ebola Rocks West Africa

In 2014 and 2015, Ebola was center stage. Named by the medieval Professor David Johnson, son of epidemiologist Karl Johnson, Ebola is characterized as a severe viral hemorrhagic fever that is easily transmissible and causes significant symptoms, including organ failure, vomiting, and diarrhea leading to death. Ebola's mortality approached 90%, initially. Ebola's high mortality

rate eventually decreased to a still lethal rate of 40% with intensive treatment measures, extreme quarantine, and social isolation steps. The high mortality rate disproportionally affected aid workers that were part of the West African response effort from the United States and Britain. The coverage of Ebola's carnage, particularly the documented human suffering, did well to promote great fear and anxiety in the disease long before many individuals in America were in genuine danger of contracting Ebola. Indeed, many experiencing the impact of Ebola, like our protagonist Dr. Mears and our ancestral Black Death brethren, felt as if this disease was different and undoubtedly akin to the end of the world. The fear of Ebola mobilized an urgent response from the global community. Pandemic fear inspired by diseases like HIV/AIDS and Ebola can be a good thing if it helps prevent unnecessary death and prepares us for the next great infectious disease calamity.

More Lessons Learned from the Black Death

Drug Resistance

The Black Death is not an immediate threat to us anymore. Although we tend not to pay it much attention, there are still invaluable lessons to be learned from this once deadly plague.

Despite effective antibiotics that can treat the plague, we must remember this ancient enemy is still around. Around the world, antibiotics, and the once heralded penicillin, are collectively losing their ability to fight disease. Pathogens, like humans, evolve. As pathogens once susceptible to our antibiotics become drug-resistant, they gain *superbug* powers by eluding our cocktail of pharmaceuticals. These mutated pathogens could present

a potential threat and become deadly once again. Perhaps the Black Death mutated to become less lethal to survive. Indeed, a pathogen like Yersinia pestis that so effectively kills off its hosts also needs to survive, and a dead host species threatens the pathogen's existence.

Small World

In 1348, before global aviation and worldwide shipping, the Genoese merchant ships sailing the Mediterranean spread the Black Plague very efficiently and effectively. The world is much smaller and far more interconnected now. Imagine how the Black Plague would have spread today. Indeed, we don't have to imagine it; we've seen it. Just look how quickly COVID-19, Severe Acute Respiratory Syndrome (SARS), and Middle East Respiratory Syndrome (MERS) spread via international flights.

Consider Ebola in our now smaller world. In October 2014, Thomas Eric Duncan traveled from Liberia to Dallas, Texas, to visit his family. Mr. Duncan became ill and was admitted to Texas Health Presbyterian Hospital. While hospitalized, he was diagnosed with Ebola and later died. Two nurses, Nina Pham and Amber Vinson, who cared for Mr. Duncan, were diagnosed with Ebola days after treating him. Before Duncan left Liberia, he had signed an affidavit to attest he had no contact with anyone known to have Ebola. It was later revealed Duncan might have provided aid to a woman in Liberia that unknowingly had Ebola. If Duncan had survived to travel back to Liberia, officials there would have reportedly taken legal action against him because of his signed affidavit. A signed piece of paper will not protect someone in one part of the world from contracting an infection in another part of the world. We are too connected, and as illustrated in the film *Contagion* and our own experience with COVID-19, ease of travel helps global pandemics travel very rapidly.

Public Health

Furthermore, the Ebola and Black Death examples highlight how the lack of a robust modern medical and public health infrastructure can exacerbate disease spread. COVID-19 demonstrated how even with a public health infrastructure in place, an epidemic could still quickly grow into a pandemic and impact countries with strong and weak political and economic systems. Like COVID-19, we observed similar missteps in the first days of Ebola's presence in the United States. Ebola illuminated that, even if the United States is ready and able to treat a disease like Ebola when outbreaks occur on US soil, our globalized, interconnected, and interdependent society provides viruses and bacteria ample opportunities to find new hosts.

Ebola is not the Black Death. Like COVID-19, Ebola is a virus. The plague is bacterial. These diseases have several other differences as well. So, what lessons could be learned from the Black Death? And why should we turn our attention away from 21st-century viral infections that have caused so much death and alarm? Why focus on a disease that seems relatively harmless when treated with antibiotics? One word answers all these questions—perspective.

Perspective from the Black Death

As Michelle Ziegler wrote in her 2014 journal article *The Black Death and the Future of the Plague*, "Sensationalizing the plague does not help us to deal with these realities, but neither does the lack of attention given to plague in areas of the world that are

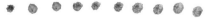

often beneath our notice."[1] Given the concerns of COVID-19, the Black Death is a disease worth our attention since it is currently classified as a re-emerging infectious disease. Armstrong and others demonstrate how the Black Death struck the world in three separate pandemics.

The Plague of Justinian in the 6th-century spread across Europe, Asia, North Africa, and Arabia like wildfire. The Black Death of the 14th-century devastated Europe. The modern 19th-century plague outbreak originated in China and spread throughout India. The outbreak in India was not readily identified because, like in many other countries, the people stopped worrying about the plague. When the infection was well established, the pathogen followed people's movements like the Black Death followed early Genoese merchant sailors. In India's case, the plague was spread by migrant workers that traveled to the city of Surat, inhabited by one and a half million people.

The migrant workers' initial infections raged through the city slums. Prime conditions for spread were close quarters, inadequate medical and public health infrastructure, and ineffective government engagement and oversight. When officials became aware of the plague's impact, over 78% of confirmed cases were determined to be in Surat's slums. Armstrong highlights the chilling parallels in Surat to the plague's natural history and presentation from the medieval world. A tipping point was reached, and the plague could not be effectively contained anymore. Medical professionals were underprepared and overwhelmed. Supplies and antibiotics were diminished, and those professionals in the hardest-hit areas could

---

[1]Michelle Ziegler, "The Black Death and the Future of the Plague," in Monica H. Green, Ed., The Medieval Globe, 1 (2014), 259–283.

no longer remain at their posts. In Surat, media headlines reported the return of the Black Death. During medieval times, the media was primitive compared to the robust apparatus of today. In the darkest days of the COVID-19 pandemic, similar reports mentioned above were promulgated across the world.

In India, the plague's news caused some people to flee to the countryside to wait out the worst of it, similar to the behavior of many during COVID-19. People were moving around a lot during a pandemic when they just should have stayed put. People migrating from Surat to Delhi and Kolkata brought the disease to others. Here, professor Armstrong again offers an especially dishearteningly familiar perspective. Members of Surat's Muslim community were falsely accused of spreading the plague through an act of bioterrorism.

Throughout the centuries, pandemic fears invariably cause some to attack the minorities among them. Indeed, in the 1980s, the ignorant and uninformed among us blamed LGBTQ individuals for HIV/AIDS. Ebola was and is still considered a Black disease. In the United States, COVID-19 was blamed on the Chinese and immigrants from Mexico and Latin America. Yes, humans have been here before. Despite over 600 years of perspective, we relive our human condition with fear and contempt again. Diseases spread, others were blamed for it, and the masses' reactions and behaviors caused further spread of the disease.

After the outbreak in Surat, the plague was discovered in Madagascar where a strain of Yersinia was alarmingly found to resist all known antibiotics used to treat the plague previously. Scientists hypothesized the Yersinia pestis bacterium borrows genetic material from other bacteria it comes in contact with (i.e., E. coli and salmonella) and then rewrites its genetic code. Through this process of lateral gene transfer, the bacterium evolves and conveys resistance to antibiotics. The lesson here is sobering and stark, and in these times of COVID-19, it's one we would all do well to heed, especially as new strains of novel coronavirus are invariably emerging.

When the plague struck India in1994, millions of people panicked. They moved when they should have stayed in place. Fortunately, despite panic, only a small number of deaths occurred. We have not been so lucky with COVID-19. Like the people in medieval Europe and modern-day India, we have not stayed in one place, isolated, or kept a social distance effectively. By the end of 2020, nearly 2 million lives were lost worldwide.

The Silver Lining

The intensive study of the Black Death, HIV/AIDS, Ebola, and other pandemics offers both instruction and perspective. A critical insight is that human beings are resilient and can and will surprise you. The Yersinia pestis bacterium showed its ability to evolve, survive, and thrive throughout the ages—so have humans. In each pandemic era, we read and encounter historical accounts about ordinary people stepping up and going to extraordinary extremes to offer help and comfort. These modern-day superheroes include our healthcare providers, first responders, essential workers, teachers, and care-givers who have humbly and sincerely performed their duties. Many have died because of their work. Leaders at all levels have tried to maintain normalcy while trying to prevent further outbreaks. Unfortunately, many ordinary people have buried children, husbands, wives, aunts, uncles, brothers, sisters, and cousins and still managed to keep going despite the loss.

In medieval times, artists and writers looked at the horrors around them and produced work that was inspired and inspiring despite the despair and grief. The artists offered social commentary and comfort to a population trying to make sense of what was happening all around them. As Armstrong and other scholars of pandemics admonish, we must not forget that without the Black Death, Italian writer Boccaccio's great works may not have emerged. Without Boccaccio, there may not have been Chaucer's *Canterbury Tales*. Chaucer, the man we call the father of English poetry, could have been a footnote in history, just someone mentioned in passing who wrote some poetry and translated some texts. Indeed, society would be much different without the pandemics that have shaped the course of human history.

In the final analysis, the vital lesson of COVID-19, Ebola, HIV/AIDS, the Black Death, and other plagues is that like those pathogens, humans, and communities do survive. We evolve, and if we are fortunate, we emerge from each pandemic and thrive. History may provide comfort. Even amid terrible despair, significant loss, and death, civilization endured. We have been here before, and many lived to tell incredible stories, and great art emerged that changed our world for the better. During COVID-19 we have seen great art emerge—and the best is yet to come.

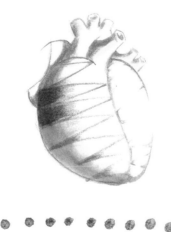

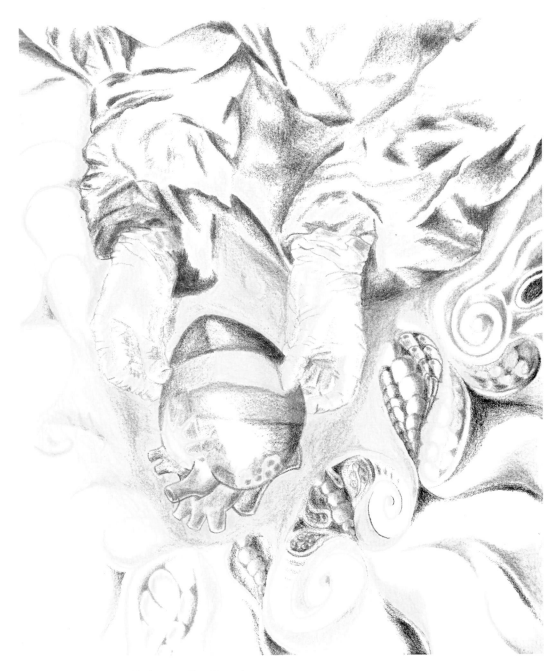

WHAT WE GIVE BACK: Understanding Sowerby

Human Care Theory

•••••••• DR. HASSAN A. TETTEH

WHAT is Human Care?

••••Human Care is timely, comprehensive care that advances each person's total health in body, mind, and spirit.

WHAT problems does Human Care address?

••••Human Care challenges the current system that is not patient-centered and that is perpetuating fragmented care, escalating costs, and inefficient delivery.

WHY is Human Care important?

••••Human Care produces a healthier society by meeting the patient's need for real care, the physician's desire to be a true healer, and the country's want of actual value for dollars spent on healthcare.

PURPOSE

••••Revive Your Healing Passion
Resurrect your commitment to the honorable and meaningful purpose of helping people feel better.

Realize Your Healing Power
Grasp the impact you make as you restore people's health so they can realize their purpose and continue the chain reaction of changing the world.

PERSONALIZATION

••••Discover Your Patient's Present
Learn your patient's current state of being, including their values, dreams, and gifts for the world.

Maximize Your Patient Encounters
Capitalize on each interaction to create trust and the respectful connection that can change the world.

PARTNERSHIP

••••Leverage Your Team Dream
Advance the collective care team effort to achieve a total health impact for all.

Shape Your Professional Horizon
Create your unique legacy to elevate and unify the healthcare community for a lasting impact on health and humanity.

CONCRETE RESULTS

••••• The antidote for burnout in healthcare.
• A new perspective on what it means to heal.
• A formula that delivers a new level of healing.
• The ideal model for providing effective care.
• A passion to make healthcare great again.

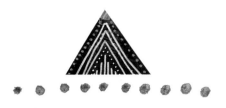

Part I

COVID-19 and Purpose

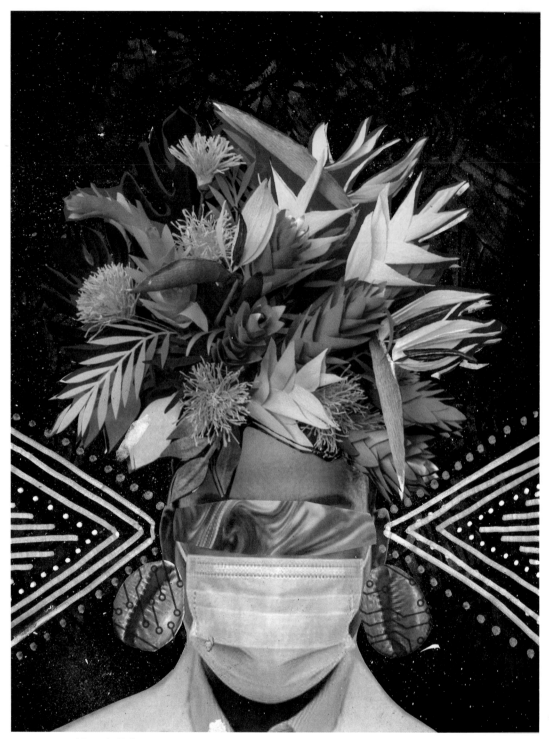

SEE NO EVIL: Massah Fofana

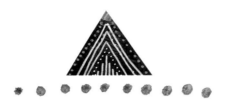

Chapter 2

My Purpose for Writing This Book

In my mind, COVID-19 started back in November 2019. I read the *Wall Street Journal*. I have it delivered every day—the paper edition. I think I get more information about medicine in the *Wall Street Journal* than any other journal because it reveals where people are spending money and factors impacting the world.

By mid-December 2019, I regularly read news about this thing called COVID-19 on the front page or below the fold every day. That's where I got my warning signal. The people who work in the markets had begun to realize that something was happening long before many of us in the health professions even understood that the novel coronavirus would be an issue.

So, back in November and then through December 2019, I started talking about COVID-19 with my colleagues from the Department of Defense Joint Artificial Intelligence Center

(JAIC) at the Pentagon. I'm one of only two doctors in the entire organization. I was telling people, "Hey, there is this COVID thing." And they'd reply, "Ah, it's just the flu." And I would say, "I don't think so. It wouldn't be getting so much attention if it was just the flu. The *Wall Street Journal* is writing about this every day."

Dr. Edward Lathan, my roommate from med school, was one of a few of my colleagues who shared my alarm. Ed is now an emergency room (ER) doctor practicing in New Rochelle, New York. He and I talk a lot. In January 2020, he told me that he had pulled his kids out of school. My reaction was, "Wow! What'd you do that for?" He said, "Hassan, something is happening. I think COVID is here."

Long before others sounded the alarms, Ed told me, "Hassan, I don't know how it's being spread. But you need to take off all your clothes and decontaminate yourself when you come home from the hospital." Ed was telling me this even before the CDC was issuing similar guidelines.

Ed also wrote a letter to the superintendent of the New Rochelle school district. He explained what he was seeing—many young people and middle-aged people coming in with very severe flu-like symptoms.

There was no testing then, but Ed thought that what he was seeing was COVID-19. He and his colleagues in the ER wrote letters, letters, and more letters, but nothing happened. So, Ed pulled his kids out of school.

March 2020: COVID-19 Changes Our Lives

In mid-March, I talked with one of my colleagues about COVID-19 when I got an alert from the *Wall Street Journal.* I said, "Hey, futures just took a hit." He was astonished.

Up until that day, nothing else I said about COVID-19 had resonated with him. I'd been talking about it for months. It took futures trading to go down substantially to pique his attention. He said, "Wait a minute. This thing is serious."

March 13, 2020, was a Friday. I recall standing outside my office around 11:00 a.m. and striking up a conversation about COVID-19 with a group of colleagues as they were heading out to lunch. They said, "Here we go again. You're talking about that flu, right?" I said, "Right. It's not the flu, but we'll see."

They went to lunch. By 4:00 that afternoon, the National Basketball Association (NBA) canceled its season. And that was the last day of 2020 that my team at the JAIC regularly came to the office. In mid-April, I received this text from one of my colleagues: "I guess you were right."

But I didn't want to be right.

As a thoracic surgeon, I see many consults in my practice. Throughout March, April, and May, I started to see many patients in the intensive care unit (ICU) with complications from COVID-19 infection: barotraumas, many chest tubes, prone ventilation, trach management, and other conditions. Then something else happened. New York became one of the places in the United States hit hardest by COVID-19. I'm from New York—a little town called Brooklyn. My hometown friends, family, and colleagues from medical school were all dealing with this extraordinary thing called COVID-19, and they were not sure what to do.

Then, I lost two aunts and an uncle to COVID-19.

I was close to my aunts and uncle. Gregory "Dad" Lewis gave me my first big break, a lifetime opportunity. He gave me my high school job at the McDonald's he managed. Why was it such an exciting opportunity? First, because I loved McDonald's back then, and I could get free food (that was one of the fringe benefits). Second, I made essential spending money for my senior trip to Disney World, which was vital for me back then.

Now, suddenly, my aunt and my uncle were not here anymore. I had an existential crisis, if you will. I had deep personal grief and dealt with the professional dilemma of seeing patients deteriorate before my eyes in a way I had never seen before.

I've taken care of some sick patients over my career. Until COVID-19, one of the sickest patients I had ever taken care of was a Burkholderia cepacia, post-lung-transplant patient. Burkholderia is an opportunistic group of complex Gram-negative bacteria that most often causes pneumonia in immunocompromised individuals with underlying lung disease. Only the most aggressive and progressive transplant centers will offer lung transplants to cepacia patients since they are very sick, sick patients. In my experience with cepacia transplant patients, I was at their bedside in the ICU for days and days and days, doing everything I could to keep them alive.

COVID-19 makes that experience look like, yes, a walk in the park. With COVID-19, I've watched patients go from one extreme to the other in a matter of moments. And what was professionally— and socially—frustrating was that a large swath of the population had not yet been impacted personally by COVID-19. They hadn't seen it. None of their family members or friends had it. If, by chance, someone they knew did have it, maybe it seemed like mild flu. To them, all the fuss made no sense. This is true, to some extent, even to this day.

Meanwhile, I was immersed in the pandemic's wake and the toll on patients. I was living it professionally. I was living it personally.

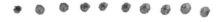

I was consumed. By April, I had emotionally descended to a shallow place. I was frustrated that what I saw on TV was so disconnected from what I saw in my own personal and professional life. I couldn't understand why people were saying that COVID-19 didn't exist, was not real, or was just made up.

In May, after a conversation with Greg Salciccioli, a brilliant man who also happens to be my executive coach and very good friend, I started to come out of my funk. He and I arranged a video conference catch-up on Zoom. I reiterate—this is a brilliant guy, an inspiring man. He coaches Fortune 100 CEOs. I had the pleasure of working with him years ago when I returned from one of my deployments. He lives in a beautiful and remote area of Oregon.

On the Zoom call, he asked, "Hey Hassan, how are you doing?"

I answered honestly. "I'm in quite a funk here, and it's because of COVID."

He replied, "This COVID thing is crazy, right? What's the big deal?"

Here was a guy I respected—not a scientist, not a physician, but a very reasonable guy, a very sharp man from whom I have learned so much—and he didn't get it? He went on to say, "Nothing's happening out here. I mean, I don't understand. Why do we have to wear masks? What's all this quarantine stuff? What's going on? I just don't get it."

I said, "Greg, what are you talking about? People are dying. Don't you see all those numbers? What do you think is happening?"

He answered, "I don't know. I don't get it."

That's when I realized it was a matter of perspective. Greg didn't share my perspective on COVID-19 yet.

That's when I decided to write this book. I know this truth. I fear we will all ultimately be impacted by COVID-19, and know that when we emerge, we will all need inspiration, instruction, and strategies to return to some normalcy and ascend to a higher place. As you may have gathered from Chapter 1, my purpose is to share my perspective on COVID-19 as a student of medical history and the pandemics of the past. My purpose is to share my view as a family member who has suffered significant loss due to COVID-19. And my purpose is, perhaps most of all, to share my perspective as a physician with knowledge gained from treating patients impacted by the current pandemic.

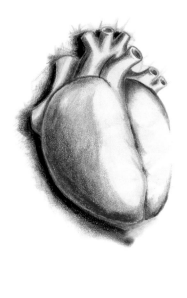

Remembering
Those We Have Lost:
Aunt Carmen

Like many people impacted by COVID-19, my family and I had to find our way back to sanity after losing loved ones to the virus. Over the 2020 holiday weekend that included Valentine's Day on Friday and Presidents' Day on Monday, our Aunt Carmen was visiting our home in Maryland. We were all sitting around the kitchen table, musing about how everyone would be back in a few months for my daughter's confirmation and, a few weeks later, for her graduation from middle school. We were discussing whether they should stay with us the whole time or go home and come back. Like aunts do, Aunt Carmen kept expressing how she couldn't believe how grown-up my daughter had become.

Carmen was my wife's aunt, and she had also worked with my mother before I was born. She had been a part of both of our families for a long time. She was the matriarch, full of energy, always providing the right words of wisdom for every situation. When I met my wife and we got married, we found it interesting that Carmen and my mother had known each other and worked together in a nursing home for many years.

Carmen loved to tell us stories about how it was for her when she was growing up and when she was in high school. She had this incredible ability to make everybody around her happy.

After she went home to New York City, we kept in touch as we realized the pandemic was beginning to hit hard there. In March, Carmen started to feel ill. We were concerned because she had underlying conditions. She had always suffered from asthma, had undergone back surgery, and was getting older. When she came down with what we thought was a cold, she went to the hospital. They kept her a few hours and released her with supportive care. Carmen felt better for a few days, but over the next few weeks, she progressively got worse.

By this time, the COVID-19 pandemic was well documented in New York City. By April, Carmen's symptoms worsened, stifling her breathing and preventing her from doing simple tasks like walking. One early evening, she was taken back to the hospital. This time, she was not released a few hours later. The hospital was not allowing family members to come in with patients, so she was admitted by herself.

In a very short time, she deteriorated. She required more and more oxygen and then had to be placed on a ventilator. All this information about her condition was coming to us in bits and pieces to our faraway place in Maryland. I tried my best to get information about her condition through friends and coworkers, without a lot of success. The hospital was overwhelmed with patients and inundated with calls.

This woman who was the matriarch of our family was now on a ventilator. We were all reflecting that it was such a tragedy for her to be unable to speak. When we were finally able to get in touch with a doctor at the hospital, we were told that things were not looking very good. It was so hard for us to receive this information, to wonder what was going through her mind while she was sedated, anxious, in pain, and on a ventilator in a hospital all by herself.

In a few days, it was clear she was doing worse, not better. We all felt helpless. We knew that she must be especially terrified because she was all by herself. One evening, a nurse arranged for a call with one of her daughters. Our cousin called us, tearful and crying, after the call. A few hours later, Aunt Carmen succumbed to COVID-19 and died.

Our cousin called us again. With a tearful, broken voice, she told us that Aunt Carmen had passed away. Then the grim reality of the situation worsened. We, her family, could not even make her funeral arrangements. The morgues were full. Carmen's body was stored in a refrigerated truck for weeks before we could finally lay her to rest.

Over the course of her time with us, Carmen was always the life of the party. Yet she died alone. To me, that was the greatest tragedy of all.

Luminate

The desire to create normalcy in the midst of uncertainty—to drop anchor away from stormy seas—is embodied in the word LUMINATE. This acronym represents a way to bring light into the experience of pandemic darkness.

LU– **Look up!** You are still alive and have another day above ground to do great things in the world.

M– **Mindfulness.** Take five minutes to pay attention to the present moment, your breathing, emotions, and thoughts; sense experiences such as taste, touch, and smells. Ground yourself. Imagine you are rooted to the Earth's core like a giant tree. Take some very deep breaths. Practice meditation or prayer. I am an avid meditator and practice Transcendental Meditation (TM).

I– **Importance.** What's important for you to get done today? Make a list, prioritize tasks, and complete those tasks, in order, one at a time. Make this list every morning when you start to work. I credit Ivy Lee, the father of American Public Relations, for this suggestion.

N– **Nurture your mind.** Every day, read or journal to maintain creative thought and nurture mental abilities. Getting lost in a good book both calms and exercises the mind. Journaling stimulates creativity, relieves stress, improves memory, and helps you set and achieve goals.

A– **Acts of kindness.** Random acts of kindness with no expectation of receiving anything in return take the focus off your problems and connect you with others—even during a pandemic. When you perform acts of kindness, you bring positivity into your world—and the universe will conspire to help you when you least expect it. "You will get all you want in life, if you help enough other people get what they want" (Zig Ziglar).

T– **Take ten thousand steps daily.** In addition to improving your physical health, exercise relieves anxiety and depression—and it's as simple as walking. I found great joy in returning to running even though the 2020 marathons I had planned to run in were canceled.

E– **Express gratitude.** I suggest writing down everything you are grateful for in a journal every day. This very beneficial exercise helps you keep track of the good things in your life, especially when the news all around you is not so good.

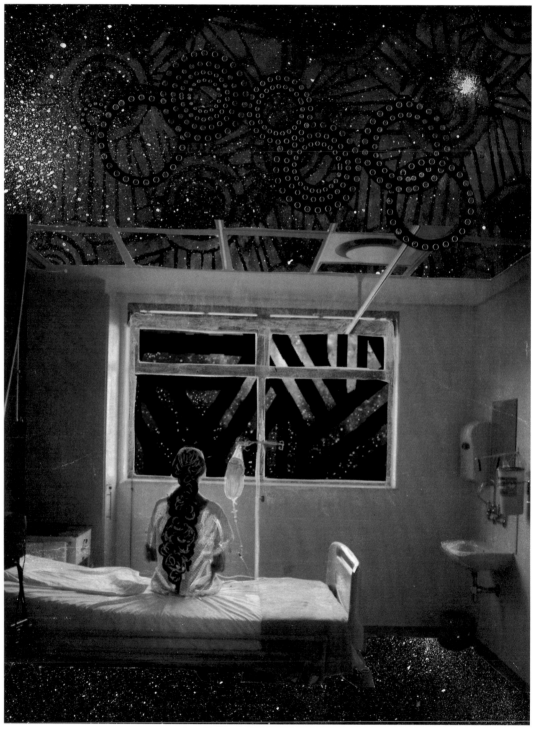

THE TREATMENT ROOM: Massah Fofana

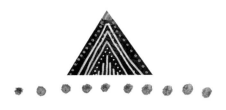

Chapter 3

Walk Out the Door as a
Different Person Than You Were
When You Came In

I invite you to have an open mind as I share with you some thoughts in this chapter. Be a little introspective! And ask yourself, "What is my purpose in life?" Maintain this question, reflect on the art, and you will emerge slightly different than when you began.

With COVID-19, we are in an unprecedented time in our world and our lives. COVID-19 has turned the world upside down. I'm a student of pandemics. I had been studying pandemics for a good long time before COVID-19 happened. I want to give you some context about this current pandemic.

I was that guy at the National War College—the only doctor in the class of 200 officers and other inter-agency people—who was always talking about the threat of viruses and bacteria. Every time I

opened my mouth, they said, "There goes that crazy doctor again." I want to think my 199 talented classmates are somewhere in the world right now saying, "Damn, that doctor was right." A little virus we can't even see with the naked eye parked an aircraft carrier and emptied the Pentagon.

Over the past year, I would argue that COVID-19 has done more harm to our national security and our country's defense than any tank, missile, or perceived threat from nuclear power.

A few years ago, I happened to be in the Mediterranean on the Greek island of Kos, not too far from Turkey. I was presenting at a conference for the World Society of Cardiothoracic Surgeons. Because it's an international meeting, they usually have it in very nice, cool places.

The Island of Kos is very small. You can literally walk around the island. I rented a bike and rode it to the site of the ancient Temple of Asclepius. Yes, it was the same temple I described in this book's introduction where Nikias received ineffective medical care. As I was standing at the site of this old temple, I thought, "That's the view, and those are the stairs that Nikias climbed."

The historical medical event that has impacted my own practice of medicine happened 2,300 years ago, right where I was standing. So here I was, a kid from Brooklyn, standing on this monument thinking, "Wow! I'm here."

On that day long ago, when Nikias met Hippocrates, he walked out the door as a different person than who he was when he came in.

As I mentioned, the island is small. And rumors spread fast there—even 2,300 years ago before Twitter and Facebook. In those days, people walked around the island (the whole island) and talked and talked.

One day, Nikias, this busy businessman, got in on the local gossip. The whole island was buzzing. "Something big is going on," thought Nikias. Then he heard the news. Someone had burned down the healing temple. Who could have done such a thing? Some scoundrel had burned down the temple. Rumors were swirling on this little island. People were talking. There was a suspect. When Nikias heard the suspect's name, he said to himself, "I know him. He's the one who took care of me. The man dressed all in white. I'll never forget his name." The scoundrel's name was Hippocrates.

And there I was, looking at the view from the top of the steps, 2,300 years later.

You're probably wondering, "What in the world does this story have to do with me?" As I said, please allow yourself an open mind for a minute. I know I can't take you to the little island of Kos and perch you where I was at the top of the temple stairs. But imagine how I must have felt being there and knowing what happened there all those years ago. Those were the steps. And this is why people like to go to the island of Hippocrates (which Kos is now known as) for medical conferences.

What does the story of Nikias and Hippocrates have to do with you in the 21st century? In the age of COVID-19? Possibly nothing, possibly a lot. But that's the question you should sear into your mind for the next few moments.

If you are a physician, ask yourself what it means to be a healer. Don't practice the kind of medicine that the priests in the temple were providing. Burn that temple down. Build a new one. No matter what your profession or calling, now is not the time to cling to what worked before March 2020. How will you respond to the changes around you? Now is the time for you to evolve.

When Nikias walked into Hippocrates' treatment room, he was sick. He was dying. His perspective was shaped by a family history that included a father and grandfather dying early deaths. Hippocrates did more than treat Nikias for chest pain that day. He changed Nikias' perspective and inspired him to make changes in his lifestyle that put him on the path to healing. Nikias did indeed walk out a different person than he was when he walked in.

What is your perspective on COVID-19? Is the fear of it paralyzing you with stress and anxiety? Is numbness wearing away at the care you provide others? Do you think it's a hoax? Please keep reading. Together, we can develop a perspective that recalls wisdom from the past, nurtures healing now, and inspires us to create a better framework for dealing with pandemics in the future. Together, we can create a purpose that fosters a new age. You, too, can walk out of COVID-19 a different person than when you walked in.

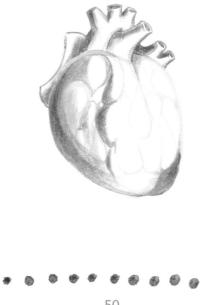

Professor Porter:
Brilliance Keeps It Simple

While I was at the Kennedy School, something unique happened. I took a class on US presidents taught by a guy named Roger Porter. It was a hard class to get into, but I got in. While I was in this class, he shared something with us that I found to be a really good way of putting things in context for so many reasons. As an economics undergrad, Porter had this great opportunity to be an intern in the Reagan administration.

If you've ever worked on Capitol Hill, and I actually had an opportunity to do that, it's really chaotic. It's not this orderly kind of thing. In fact, if you want to see a show that I think encapsulates the Hill's culture, it's that TV comedy show Veep. *That's really how it is. It's crazy. No one knows what's going on. It's all a big craziness.*

When he was an intern, Professor Porter was milling around on the West Wing when the White House Chief of Staff came out, looked around, and called out, "Hey you, Roger, come here. Listen, you're an economics major, right? You know something about economics?" Porter said yes. The chief of staff said, "Good. You've got to brief the president right now."

Reagan was about to have an interview with a newspaper about US/Russian economic policy. So, Porter gets pulled into the Oval Office. He's sitting there with the chief of staff. The president's about to come in. Reagan is about to be briefed by an undergrad. Porter's sitting there with the chief of staff. President Reagan comes in. The chief of staff says, "Mr. President, we know you have a brief in a few minutes. We brought our foremost expert on US/Russian economic policy to brief you, to tell you all you need to know."

As Professor Porter gets to this part of the story, we students are all on the edge of our seats, wondering what's going to happen next. The professor continued, "I'm sitting there and there's a silence, right? A pregnant pause—everyone's looking at me, the foremost expert, the undergrad in economics. And I say, 'Mr. President, there are only three things you need to know about US/Russian economic policy.'" Then Porter proceeded to break down his understanding of that policy into three, graspable points.

If you look up Roger Porter's career after his undergrad, intern experience as the foremost expert in US/Russian economic policy, you will find that he served as a senior advisor to President George H. W. Bush, became a member of the National Economic Council, *and went on to have a lot of good things happen for him, including becoming a professor at Harvard.*

His point in telling us this story was that anybody can take something that's really complicated and make it more complicated. That requires no mental energy. You don't even need a brain cell to do that. You can take anything and make it more complicated. But genius takes something complicated and makes it simple. That's what he was illustrating. That was the lesson he seared into my mind. And that was the brilliance of his story and his career.

When I am sharing something complicated, I always try to not make it more complicated. I recognize that there's no brilliance there. But to take something really complicated and make it simple is really good for human care—purpose, personalization, and partnerships.

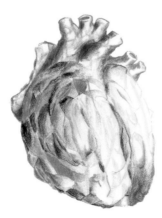

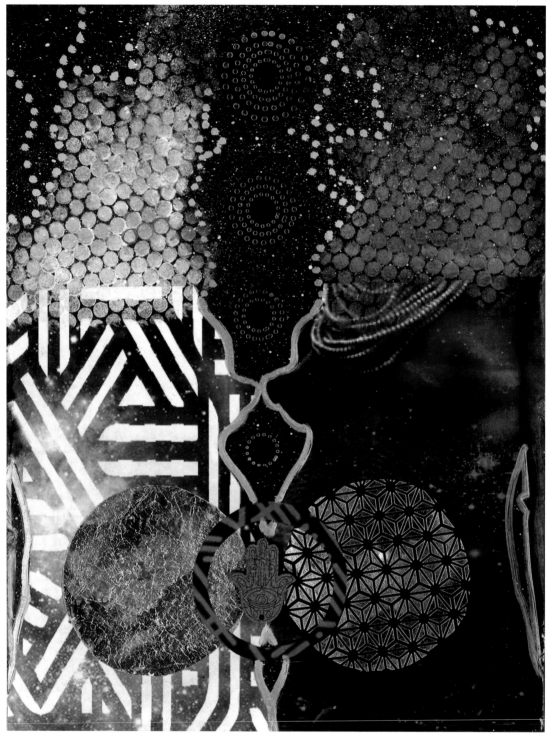

PURPOSE INSPIRES: Massah Fofana

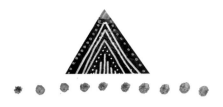

Chapter 4

What Is *Your* Purpose?

Every day I'm reminded of how precious life is.

Each day in my practice, I experience the tragic loss of organ donor patients. I also share this incredible miracle of life on the other side when someone receives a new organ.

It's a constant reminder of the delicate balance between life and death. But more importantly, it reminds us that when you have health, energy, and vitality, the entire world is open to you. If you wake up each new day with that perspective, you have the incredible power to accomplish anything your heart and mind set out to do.

To me, transplant medicine embodies the total package of healthcare. It's a very comprehensive, very professionalized, and very caring and nurturing kind of practice. And this includes

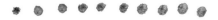

transplants for all organs, whether it be kidneys, liver, heart, lung—all of them.

When we evaluate patients for transplant, one of the things we do is assess. We want to make sure the person is going to do well. For instance, many people who need a liver transplant have self-inflicted cirrhosis. They have been drinking too much alcohol. We have to make sure the patient who receives this gift is not going to drink again, that they have changed their life—that they have developed a new purpose. It's the same way with lung transplant patients who were smokers. They must stop smoking—forever.

We also make sure the patient has a social network and support system in place. We make sure they have family members they can rely on when they need help getting to appointments or taking medications.

Foundational in transplant evaluations is *purpose.* When we evaluate a patient for transplant, we look at all aspects of their life: physical, emotional, and spiritual. We want to make sure that transplant is the right therapy for them and that they're going to do well with this gift of life. If you can get a patient to think about what their purpose is and what they want to be living for, that's the first critical step to recovery.

The purpose is fundamental. It's not the kind of thing where you wake up one day and say, "Ah, this is my purpose." Almost always, it is in the act of doing something for others that you discover your purpose.

Purpose Inspires Human Care

During my deployments to Afghanistan, purpose drove my medical team to accomplish impossible medical feats in the middle

of a war-torn desert. We were all medical people, not soldiers. Yet we all carried weapons since we were in a bad neighborhood. We were deployed with the Marines—doctors, nurses, corpsmen, and surgeons. We were in the middle of a desert with no plumbing and no electricity, only generators.

We were there during a time when the II Marine Expeditionary Force was experiencing significant casualties. Warfighters were stepping on IEDs and getting blown up. I thought I was an excellent surgeon. I trained in Brooklyn, Kings County. I had seen gunshot wounds. I did major trauma cases and saved lives. I did Whipples (pancreaticoduodenectomies). I had done everything, or so I thought. As a cardiac surgeon, I thought I had seen it all.

Then I went to Afghanistan. Imagine seeing arms, legs, scrotums gone and blown away, leaving torsos still intact because of the flak jackets. When wounded soldiers arrived with a pulse and signs of life, every one of them who came to our mobile surgical hospital tent went out alive. If they came into our tent with vital signs, we stabilized them, and they moved on to the next round of care. In the seven months I was out there, we never lost a patient.

I'm proud to say that the credit went to our team. None of us knew each other before we went on the deployment, but we made it work. I lived in tents with some of the world's most eccentric people, but I loved them to death because of the amazing things we did in the middle of nowhere. I believe the injuries we saw and treated in the desert would not have survived even in the best trauma centers today. I would measure us against any one of those centers and say we would outperform them— and with no electricity, a meager operating room, and a walking blood bank.

When I say a walking blood bank, I mean that when traumas came in, we pulled blood from people who walked into the operating room and gave it immediately to the wounded. Everyone knew their blood type. This practice taught us something. Whole blood is a lot more useful than bank blood. It has all the platelets, plasma, and other factors that work better for treating trauma in the face of massive bleeding.

We did things every day that defied possibilities. When I returned stateside and sat in meetings with my colleagues and listened to bickering, office politics, and petty stuff going on, I thought to myself, "We don't have enough urgency. Our problems are not big enough."

When you have a real purpose, it's amazing how people rally together. Whenever someone came to see us in our tent in Afghanistan, we had an urgent purpose—to keep them alive. They would die unless we did something. The medical team put petty grievances aside and figured out what that "something" was. Because we had a purpose, we made the impossible possible every day in the desert.

COVID-19 is collectively giving us a purpose. The crisis helped us all reassess what was most important in our lives. For many, it was friends and family—and hunkering down and staying safe together. Many people lost their jobs and had to reinvent themselves. How? By rediscovering their purpose. With COVID-19 among us, we all might feel pretty much the same way my team felt while performing life-or-death surgeries in a tent in the middle of a war-torn desert. Purpose got us through. Find your purpose during this pandemic, and you will find the lifeline that gets you through and helps you be the change the world needs today.

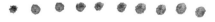

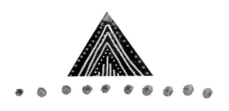

Part II

COVID-19
and Personalization

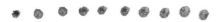

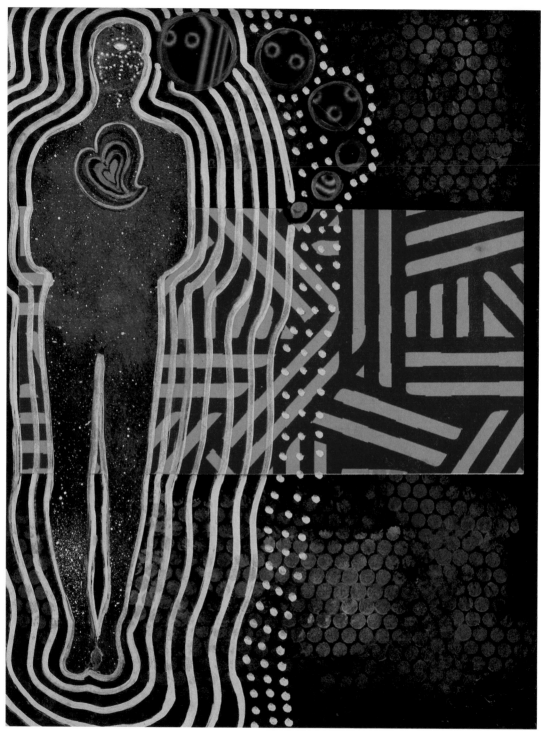

PANDEMIC STRESS: Massah Fofana

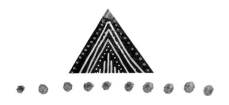

Chapter 5

My Battle with COVID-19

As I mentioned in Chapter 2, I was immersed in the COVID-19 pandemic professionally and personally. Two of my aunts and an uncle died, and I was treating patients in the hospital every day. Simultaneously, I was running into smart people who told me COVID didn't exist, and I struggled with how to reconcile this.

In 2019, I wrote and released a book, *The Art of Human Care.* I had this massive plan to roll it out in 2020. I was invited to a local venue, Busboys and Poets, to be a featured open mic artist. This invitation was such an honor for me. Many years ago, after writing my first book, *Gifts of the Heart,* I tried and tried and failed to be invited to that establishment. On January 1, 2020, I was the featured artist at Busboys and Poets, and my new book was on sale there. I knew it—2020 was going to be one of the most consequential years of my life.

I had plans to share the book at meetings and provide copies of the book to students, face-to-face, at many medical school commencements where I was invited as the keynote speaker. I had a grand plan. I thought, "I'm going to influence the next generation of doctors and nurses. This experience is going to be awesome."

Another of my exciting goals for the year was running in the 2020 Boston Marathon and the 2020 New York Marathon. However, soon after my great debut at Busboys and Poets, February came along, and I became more aware of how severe this COVID-19 pandemic would be and how it would impact society. I stopped training because I knew there was no way in the world that those marathons would happen. This pandemic was coming. What was the purpose of training? So I stopped running altogether.

Then COVID-19 hit. Everything shut down. The talks I had lined up through September 2020 were all canceled. (Zoom is not the same as doing it in person.) I became depressed. I thought, "What am I going to do?"

COVID-19 had hit me deep down and personal. It put me in a dark cloud. Some of my loved ones had died. It was hard going to work every day. My friends were getting laid off—physicians were getting laid off. How could that happen? How could you lay off a physician in the middle of a pandemic? My wife got laid off. She's a nurse at my children's school. All of this difficulty was happening all around. And I took it personally.

How do you get out of a funk if you happen to be in one? Indeed, everyone's going to be different. Like most people impacted by the virus, I recognized that I was having a serious, personal mental health challenge.

Following My Own Advice

One morning in May, I realized that many of the things I had espoused in my book were personally relevant. I remembered my own three Ps: Purpose, Personalization, and Partnerships—and finding purpose would be my first step. My purpose became to make the most of the quarantine. I started small. I decided I needed a new routine to replace the one I had lost. On May 15, 2020, I began running again, at least a mile every day. That was my genesis of reemerging from that COVID-19 funk. Running has been great for me. For one, it's given me a regimen.

For many of us, especially those who began working at home during this pandemic, we didn't even have to change clothes. We didn't have to practice hygiene. We stayed in our sweats all day, walked around, ate food, watched TV, and got on the phone. If someone stopped to ask, "What day is it? What time is it?" we would genuinely offer, "I don't know."

So I started running to get back into a routine. I got up in the morning. I ran. This practice helped my brain register that today is different than yesterday. Today is a new day.

COVID-19 also forced many of us to spend more time with our immediate families. Even though quarantine was challenging, it also was uniquely rewarding. We were at home together and didn't kill each other. We started to get to know each other better. For example, my son started telling me about what he learned in the chemistry class he had taken the past summer—that was a fascinating change in our relationship!

Another significant change for us was the puppy our daughter convinced us to get her. My wife and I were convinced it would be the worst thing in the world to do. We knew it would be like having

another child. We resisted for a long time. We finally surrendered, and we got her the puppy. That little furball, our precious Chloe, has distracted my daughter (and the rest of us) from the pandemic's daily chaos. We realized our daughter's bond with Chloe was needed to help her through quarantine, something to step in for all of her lost social opportunities. She is absolutely in love with Chloe. She has a pal to spend hours and hours with. She plays with her and is responsible for taking her for walks. They are inseparable.

COVID-19 inspired my family to take a personal inventory, to do some family housekeeping. Whether we were ready or not, change happened. We found each other. We adjusted. We evolved.

This human care theory of mine came about through a series of fascinating, personal experiences that happened in my life as a patient, as a practicing physician, and through my many patients' studies and observations. I think I've learned more from my patients than I've learned from anybody else. It was time for me to remember all I had learned.

Through a lot of introspection, good friends, support, and saying to myself, "Wait a minute. How am I personally going to get through this pandemic?" I managed to see my way out of that fog.

Politically, economically, socially, and technologically, COVID-19 will fundamentally change our society. Whenever you hear someone say, "I can't wait until we go back to normal," know that they are not living in the real world. There's no such thing as going back to normal. Let me be clear. There's no such thing as going back to normal.

No one's life is going to go back to the way it was before March 13, 2020. March 2020 was a milestone, a goal post. This "return to normal" is a fallacy.

But it also is an opportunity.

Take inventory. What is your reason for living? Who are the people who mean the most to you? What is the best way for you to deal with pandemic stress? Figure out what those things are. And don't be surprised if the person you were going into the pandemic looks a lot different from the person who confidently steps out.

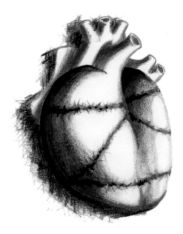

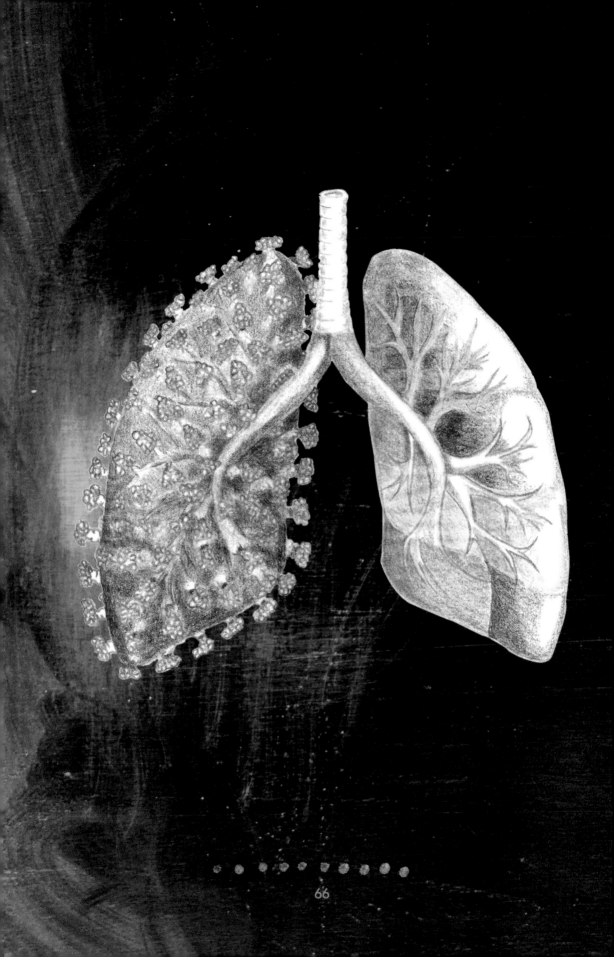

COVID-19
Up Close and Personal

Shortly after COVID-19 began infecting people here in the United States, I was assigned a transplant recovery case. Due to the tragedy of another, we were given the opportunity to recover a healthy pair of lungs for a very sick patient on the transplant waiting list. The donor had been hospitalized several days before he died. And the hospital had admitted many COVID-19 patients. While many hospitals were not testing transplant donors for COVID-19 at this point in the pandemic, this patient had been tested, and tested negative. Sadly, this must have been a case where that negative was false.

When we got our first look at the lungs, we did an evaluation, and they looked fine. They were a nice pink and had that typical healthy, spongy texture. As we progressed through the recovery, the lungs began turning gray. By the time we were ready to remove them—organ recovery of this sort takes about two hours—the lungs had completely turned to a dark, blotchy gray and took on a tough, fibrous texture.

I believe that what I was witnessing, in a very up-close and personal way, was COVID-19 ravaging the lungs in real time. This was another instance of my professional personalization with COVID-19.

I had never in all my years seen such rapid and complete deterioration of organs during the recovery process. We realized these lungs, which had been pink and healthy less than two hours before, had become so severely damaged that we had to quickly pivot to salvage other organs. Sadly, we were not able to bring new lungs to the waiting transplant patient. I never learned if that person lived to receive another pair of lungs for transplant.

As I watched this horrible scene unfold, I understood how patients, like my Aunt Carmen, could be one minute just a little short of breath and the next, gasping for air.

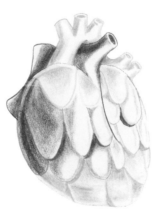

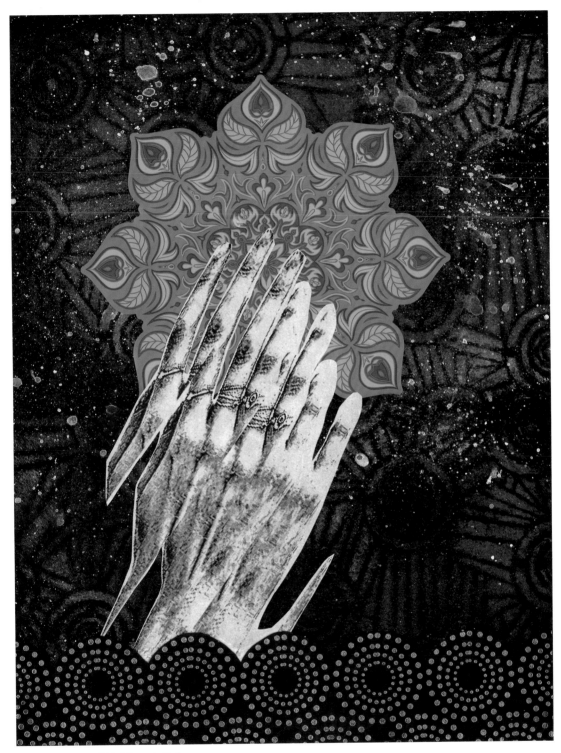

GRANDMA'S HANDS: Massah Fofana

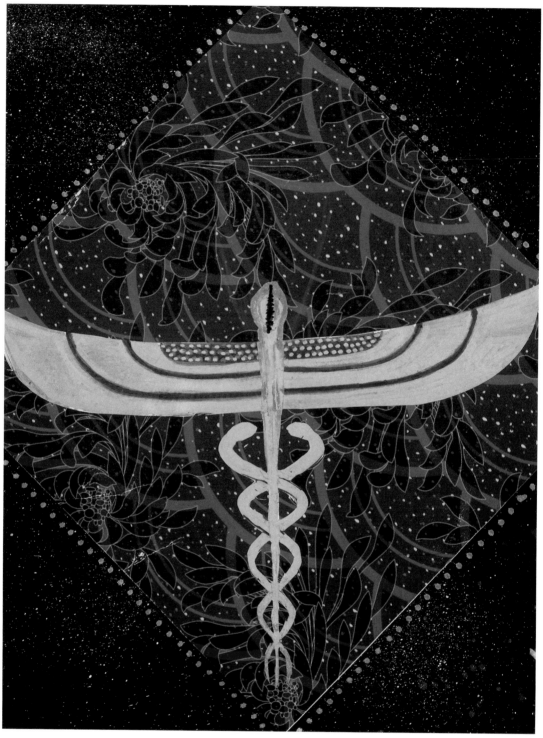

RESPONSIVE TO CHANGE: Massah Fofana

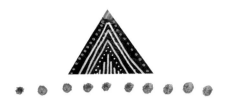

Chapter 6

Be Responsive to Change, New Opportunities

Clearly, since COVID-19, our world is on a different trajectory. People are afraid to go out. No one wants to touch each other. In my studies about past plagues and pandemics, I've uncovered behaviors that have endured to impact societal and cultural norms permanently. For instance, one theory purports that individuals from Eastern civilizations avoid social touching and hugging because several pandemics originated there.

During past plagues, people realized they didn't survive too long when they were touchy-feely and huggy-kissy. Instead, they substituted bowing and saying hello. Perhaps these behavior patterns evolved to ensure survival. Darwin didn't say "survival of the fittest" but rather the survival of those most responsive to change.

So here's your moment. Be responsive to change. If you haven't figured out that the world has changed yet, I'm here to tell you that it has.

Find Your Purpose, and You Will Discover How to Evolve

What do you love? I love to help people. I love to operate. I love recovering an organ and seeing someone with heart failure or end-stage lung disease get that new organ. And I love seeing them the next day, extubated, breathing on their own, when they look like a brand-new person. Nothing brings me more joy. That amazing feeling is unparalleled. That is my mission.

Most of us went into our professions with a mission. That mission may have gone wayward over time—we get beat up. I did.

Friends and colleagues warned me about the challenges of managing a team of surgeons and medical professionals and stressed that it wasn't something I should strive for. Yet COVID-19 forced me to change and evolve; it required responsiveness. It wasn't easy, and it was very challenging. However, I have to do what I have to do in order to do the thing I love—my vocation, my calling. Our work in transplant is something the world needs because there's undoubtedly a long list of people waiting for transplants.

I'm not suggesting that we should live one-dimensional lives. We're all multi-dimensional.

When the COVID-19 pandemic hit, I never imagined we could persuade cardiac surgeons to trust other cardiac surgeons, like our Specialized Thoracic Adapted Recovery (STAR) Team, to recover the hearts and lungs they needed for their patients.

When I presented this idea before the pandemic at the plenary session of the International Society of Heart and Lung Transplantation in 2019, many saw it as an impossible concept and asked endless questions. "How do you get the doctors to trust you? How does this practice work? How do you get reimbursed?" And I did not have all the answers at the time. I was still trying to figure all of that out.

What I did have was another colleague on the West Coast who was doing what I was doing with my STAR Team. Together and over 10 years, we had amassed over 1,000 heart and lung organ recoveries between the two of us—not a small number considering that most large transplant centers only do 30 to 40 heart and lung transplants per year.

Even so, the audience expressed much uncertainty, questioning, and hesitancy. COVID-19 reversed all that doubt. It made our concept much more comfortable to accept.

Before the pandemic, we had patients coming into the hospital, traveling for hours, often many miles all this way—like Nikias. They had chest pain. They had to wait maybe a month to get in for their appointment. They had to walk a mile to get to the doctor's office once inside the hospital center and then sit in the office for another hour. Because of pandemic-inspired regulatory changes allowing telemedicine services to be reimbursed, patients no longer have to travel great distances and wait all that time. They can stay home and visit their doctors via a video-call. In many cases, their doctors can prescribe treatment or medication over the phone. Do we want to go back to all that unnecessary waiting, traveling, and more waiting?

Opportunity is knocking. Think about places like Washington, DC, Maryland, Virginia, Atlanta, Chicago, New York City, Los Angeles—all those people getting in their cars every day. They commute two hours this way and two hours that way to work in an office next to people they might not even like, talk to people they don't want to talk to, and sit in meetings that seem to hamper their productivity. They can't even get their work done because there are so many interruptions.

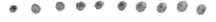

Because of COVID-19, many of us can now be at home and do all the work we want. We can Zoom, talk to the people we want to talk to, and text them if we don't feel like having a conversation. How are you going to get those people to go back to that old way? It's going to be hard.

Technology has enabled us to respond to the changes that COVID-19 has imposed upon us. In the past, no one had a choice. We had to go to the office because that was where all the stuff was. The copy machine was there. The computer was there.

This time is a new era. You don't have to do that, so evolve.

What Are Your New and Unique Opportunities?

Because of COVID-19, we all have unique opportunities to understand our workplaces' challenges, our disciplines, and our fields. You can't read leadership theory and apply it carte blanche to any situation because that's not how the world works. Everybody's problem is different.

For example, I wouldn't go to Wisconsin and tell doctors to do things exactly how we do them in Virginia, Maryland, and Washington, DC. I don't know what is happening in Wisconsin. Instead, I could give them some framework, ask them to think about how they could personalize this or that concept, or present my theory. It takes understanding your specific situation and examining it on a personal level—for yourself and for those with whom you engage.

Do you want to be distinguished from your peers? Think of a particular way to personally address a problem or take care of a situation, using the perspective that only you have. You will be invaluable.

Remembering Those We Have Lost: More Than Two Million Souls

Our world will never be the same. We lost more than 2.3 million souls globally to COVID-19 and more than 450,000 in the United States alone. In previous chapters, I shared that pandemics change the world. With the departure of the many we lost, there is a void. The emptiness is the reason our world is different. COVID-19 dimmed the light of each soul prematurely and rapidly.

As we emerge from our shelter-in-place and exchange correspondence with our social networks again, we will realize how significant our loss, indeed, has been. You will hear a familiar refrain: "Wow! I had no idea that he had COVID-19." And others will report, "I can't believe she died from COVID-19." And still others will find a reason and cause to extend their condolences to their friends and colleagues who lost loved ones to COVID-19.

Those We Lost

We have lost mothers and fathers, brothers and sisters, sons and daughters, uncles and aunts, nieces and nephews, and cousins. Families have changed. Early in the pandemic, I learned of one young lady in New York City who lost 10 family members to COVID-19. How can that be reconciled? How can one manage so much grief? How can one have hope after such a loss? Indeed, these were the same questions the people of Athens asked during the plague as they questioned God's existence and the same question the families of the Black Death asked. At the turn of the 20th century, many wondered how they could continue to live on in the face of the Spanish Flu. Yet through all those pandemics, humans survived, adapted, and continued. Faith was restored, art emerged, healing occurred, and resilience allowed us to recover from each threat and prepare to face the next disease.

Those Who Survived

For those who recover from COVID-19, there will forever be a remembrance and, ideally, a sense of gratitude for survival. This experience engenders necessary reflection. My transplant work reminds me of how fragile life is. The awareness of how each day is a gift can be remarkably empowering. For those who embrace the experience of dodging death as a gift, a new world perspective is a result. You can place past failures, challenges, and difficulties behind you. You can begin to assess your days ahead with freshness. What changes should you make? What new path should you chart? What opportunities should you explore? It is possible, however, as a survivor to miss this opportunity for renewal. Here is where we must remember those we have lost. In the more than two million lives lost, think about how many dreams were unfulfilled, how many birthdays went uncelebrated, how many trips were not traveled, how many goals deferred, how many languages not learned, and how many relationships not started or improved.

The Way Ahead for Those Who Remain

We must honor those we lost by celebrating each day as a gift. As we emerge from COVID-19's threat, remember how our ancestors demonstrated that each pandemic created the opportunity for human growth. The Renaissance, the Enlightenment, and the Roaring Twenties illustrate the human spirit with brilliance and serve as a potential blueprint for this moment. Be a light. When there is light there is hope. Luminate with more extraordinary brilliance and work to replace the void left by the departure of those we lost. Now is the opportunity to rediscover your purpose. Personalize the moment, and partner with others to bring about a change.

How Will You Be Remembered?

Will people remember that you had a long and successful career? As they remember you, will they recount your place of birth, the schools you attended, and your contributions? Who will they say you helped, and what service will you be remembered for? Will you pioneer new advances that endure? Did you solve problems to make life easier for others? Will your friends and professional colleagues recognize you with awards, honors, and acclaim? Will you teach *others? Will people remember you for your mentorship and the wisdom you imparted to others? What art will you leave behind? How will you lift the spirit of others? Will it be with poetry, painting, sculpture, dance, photography, or the words you write? Who will survive you? How will your family remember you? What will they report to others when you are gone? Will you be gone and not forgotten, or will you be forgotten but not gone?*

Use this pandemic as a moment of change and growth. Remember those we lost. Work on your destiny now so your legacy ensures you will be admired for what you do, respected for what you say, and remembered for what you write.

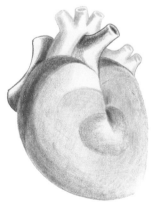

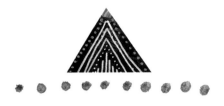

Part III

COVID-19
and Partnerships

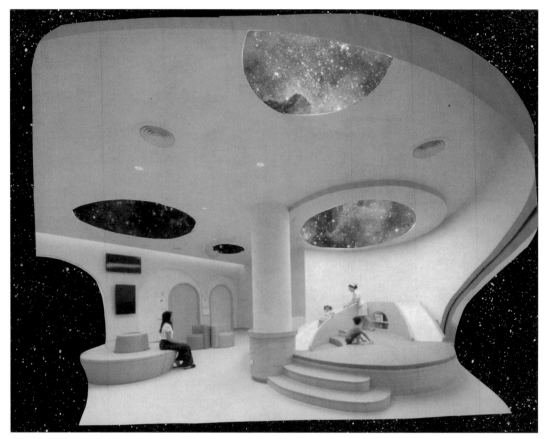

HEALTHCARE REVOLUTION: Massah Fofana

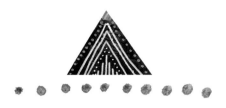

Chapter 7

COVID-19, Transplants, and Partnerships

When COVID-19 came along, all our elective cardiac cases stopped. Overburdened hospitals postponed elective procedures. Sick people were not going to the hospital because they feared they would catch the disease there. I shared with my colleagues, "We have a practice where we recover hearts and lungs for transplantation for desperately ill patients in need. I'm not sure if COVID is going to hurt us or help us."

What happened was surprising. An enormous amount of opportunity evolved from the pandemic. COVID-19 shifted and altered the transplant landscape. In early 2019, based on over a decade of research, I shared a model at the International Society for Heart and Lung Transplantation (ISHLT) called Specialized Thoracic Adapted Recovery (STAR) Teams. The model demonstrated how

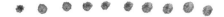

heart and lung organs, typically subject to short, cold, ischemic times of four to six hours, could be recovered like the abdominal organs. Ischemic time is the time between cross-clamping, the interruption of blood flow to the donor's heart or lungs, and the reperfusion, reestablishing blood flow of the donor's heart and lungs in the recipient.

This interval is critical for heart and lung transplantation because ischemic injury beyond maximal limits occurs to the heart and lungs because of lack of perfusion and oxygen to the donated organ cells. Here is how the geography of transplant works. Local transplant surgeons usually recover the abdominal organs when a donor becomes available. A doctor in Ohio may recover a liver and send it by courier for a patient in Kansas. Recovered livers and kidneys last longer than hearts and lungs, substantially longer. They have cold ischemic times of 12 to 48 hours.

In practice and traditionally, heart and lung transplant surgeons seldom, if ever, allow local teams of cardiac surgeons to recover those donated organs. Trusting their team exclusively, heart and lung transplant centers send their own surgeons to recover donated hearts and lungs.

However, COVID-19 blew up that whole paradigm. To prevent the spread of COVID-19 in the Washington, DC region, hospital centers did not permit transplant teams from other locations to travel to their hospitals, especially during the spring and summer of 2020, if they were coming from areas where COVID-19 was prevalent.

Left with limited options, the heart and lung transplant centers allowed local surgeons and our STAR team, in particular, to recover heart and lung organs. During those initial months of the pandemic, we recovered well over 25 donated heart and lung

organs, developed excellent relationships and trust with transplant centers nationwide, and saved the lives of desperately ill patients who may not have survived without a new heart or lungs.

The transplant centers partnered with our team and adopted the STAR Team model. Our STAR Team has been in place for more than 12 years and has worked well to increase the number of heart and lung transplant cases, improve patient outcomes, and reduce the cost associated with transplantation. Our STAR team has become central to my clinical practice. Given the irregular hours and spontaneity of cases, recovering heart and lung organs is demanding, yet it is also gratifying. Donor organ recoveries usually happen outside of regular office hours, at night, and on weekends.

Over time, we noticed our STAR Team practice helped transplant centers, especially during the COVID-19 pandemic, by providing an invaluable service that otherwise required the attention of a full-time surgical employee. Our STAR Team's group of surgeons and professional staff allowed the recipient transplant center surgeons to avoid canceling scheduled elective surgeries and focus on the transplant recipient patient's needs. Using our STAR Team also meant that hospitals didn't have tired, disgruntled surgeons who had been up all night now operating on their ill recipient patient. We alleviated that burden for them. I would never have anticipated that a pandemic such as COVID-19 would provide the opportunity for sharing the benefits of STAR Teams and help us evangelize the benefits of a model developed over a decade of dedicated practice.

COVID-19 has swung other pendulums of medical practice in positive new directions and ushered in additional paradigm changes. I was talking to one of my colleagues about telemedicine.

She shared, "I don't have to go to the hospital. I'm talking to all my patients. I'm prescribing things. I'm helping them. I have more time with them. Who would have known, right?"

Developing these positive steps took an evolution of thought. We could have sat there in our funk and thought, "Oh, this is the worst thing ever. The world's coming to an end."

COVID-19 has also unmasked the urgent need for us to make other changes in our world. Consider the vast businesses, the flagship companies, and the brands that have gone bankrupt since COVID-19 hit. How is that possible? How could, for example, Century 21, Chuck E. Cheese, Briggs & Stratton, Lord & Taylor, and Brooks Brothers go out of business? These were iconic companies.

Suppose you look at the history of businesses at any given time, whether during a boom, bust, or in between. A company's failure usually exposes what already was an underlying problem. Crisis accelerates impending demise. Chances are, if we had waited another 10 or 20 years, all those companies might have folded anyway. The change was coming, with or without COVID-19. Pandemics accelerate the changes society will face.

For example, look how we are living now. People live in sweats and casual attire! We don't need suits, at least not right now. I love suits. However, maybe we were all tired of wearing suits anyway. If Brooks Brothers had figured that out, they might have adapted and offered a classic fashion for the times we live in. Crisis forces change faster. If we don't evolve, we don't survive.

COVID-19 exposed institutional structural issues and problems in these companies that accelerated their failure. If this pandemic hadn't hit, they might have had more time to figure out something different. But COVID-19 came. And change came.

Wherever you are in your life, whether you are an emergency room physician, an ICU nurse, a caregiver for elderly parents, a schoolteacher, or a first responder, think about what you were doing before March 2020. Please realize that we are not going back to that. Then ask yourself, "What can I do for my department, my patients, my team, my students, my family—what can I do for myself right now? How do I evolve? Do I need to learn some new skills? Do I need to do something differently? What new partnerships should I build?"

Look forward and beyond. Our society isn't going to come out of the door the same as it was when it went in. How can we come out better together?

It's true. The world is always changing. COVID-19 has caused the world to change faster. Like with pandemics of the past, COVID-19 has forced us to evolve and adapt more quickly. All of us who survive COVID-19 need to figure out how we will grow into our next phase. We have to create our new normal. We must negotiate our shared existential crisis.

What will our next renaissance look like? That is up to us.

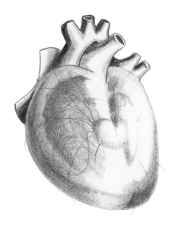

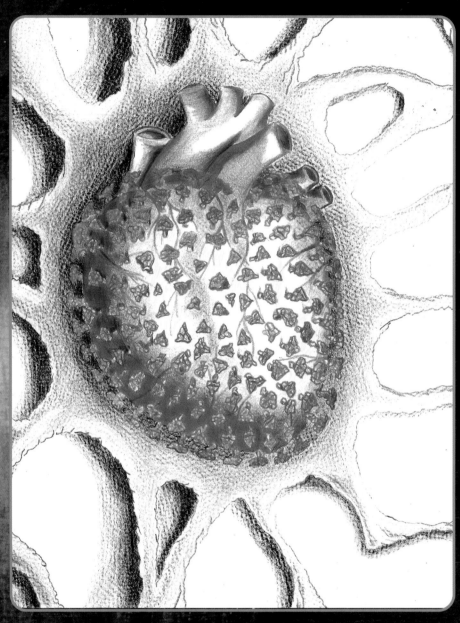

COVID-19 HEART: Understanding Sowerby

How Ebola Set
the Stage

In July 2015, I had the opportunity to go to work in my father's birth country, Ghana—not to visit family but to join West Africa's fight against Ebola. My role in the West Africa Disaster Preparedness Initiative was to develop a curriculum and teach about crisis communications in Ghana, Togo, and Senegal. My colleagues from the U.S. Army, U.S. Air Force, and I joined local experts to facilitate an Ebola Awareness Course to guide response to the epidemic.

Together, we developed a framework for the course, the 3Ws, to address those at risk for the disease. The goal was to instill confidence, share accurate information, and inspire behaviors that lowered the pandemic's risks. This framework helped dispel the kinds of misinformation and outlandish falsehoods that frightened people tend to grasp onto when faced with highly contagious diseases. If you are aware of how misinformation heightened the risks of COVID-19 here in the United States, you understand the importance of our work there.

The 3Ws asked, "What happened? What are you doing about it? What does it mean to me?" The World Health Organization (WHO) and the Centers for Disease Control and Prevention (CDC) regularly highlighted "what" was happening, "what" was being done, and "what" the crisis meant to individuals.

Since the initial 2014 reports in Guinea, thousands of individuals, including members of the US military, and billions of dollars in resources were mobilized to address the Ebola outbreak, contain its spread, and treat the sick directly impacted by the deadly virus. For those who had been leading the fight against Ebola, the 3Ws provided a practical checklist for rapidly and effectively communicating during the crisis.

When the WHO identified COVID-19 as a global pandemic in early March 2020, world leaders had to rapidly communicate their plans to mitigate its dangers and save lives. The same 3Ws framework can help communicate that COVID-19 is worse than other infections. And it can help explain the efficacy of preventive measures to contain the spread of infection; for example, masks, hand washing, and body temperature screening.

I realized that we in America were missing some opportunities to be more effective in the ways we communicated what was happening with COVID-19. Thankfully, we've made some changes that may have helped save lives.

How a message is successfully delivered during a crisis is very critical to whether or not lives are saved. Without the partnerships forged in West Africa to fight Ebola, that pandemic would no doubt have had even higher death tolls. And those partnerships—and the invaluable models for crisis communication they created—can be an important force in shaping continued responses to COVID-19 and future pandemics.

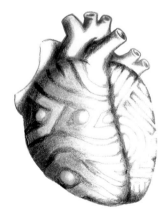

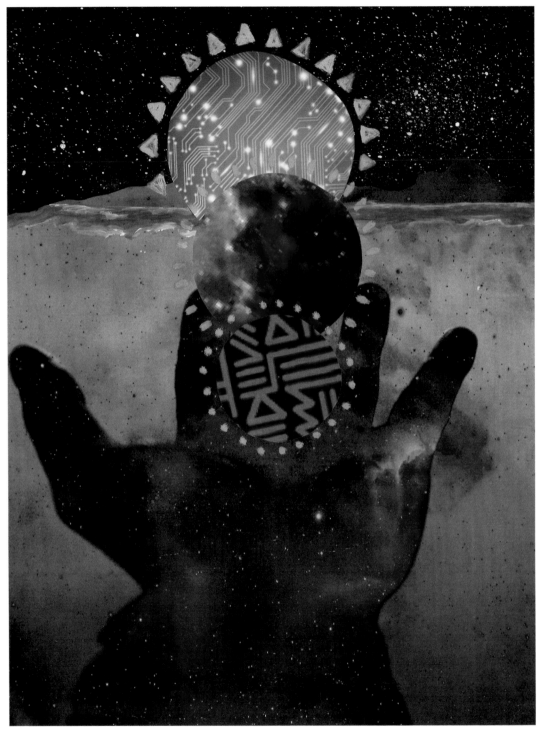

MAGIC HAPPENING: Massah Fofana

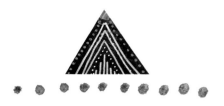

Chapter 8

There's a Magic Happening

I am rededicating my mission, if you will, to getting this message out, especially during this time of COVID-19. I began partnering with people, many people, to deliver a message that I hope will be helpful and inspirational, and if nothing else, bring some art into the world that will bring a smile to people's faces and lift their souls.

During 2020, you could not go anywhere and not think about COVID-19. This pandemic continues to impact every aspect of our lives in 2021. Perhaps you have experienced it firsthand—you've heard about somebody you know who's been sick, or you have been ill. Even if you've only been watching it on the news, have never seen a case of it, and don't know what all the fuss is about, it has, at the very least, impacted your life. Everyone—in America anyway—remembers where they were in mid-March 2020. A cascade of events led us to live in a vastly different world.

Very early on, like many people, I felt dispassionate about everything. It was hard. I couldn't go to work. I couldn't meet with my team members. I wasn't doing my daily routine. I started to have family members who were hospitalized.

As I was taking care of patients with complications of COVID-19, I felt like I was having an existential, out-of-body experience. I knew so much about pandemics. I learned how bad they were. But now, one was impacting me. Personally. Professionally. My son had started his freshman year of high school. Then the whole second half of his year was devastated, just as he was finding his stride in sports, academics, and friendships. My daughter was graduating from middle school. She was going to celebrate the sacrament of confirmation and prepare for graduation. The very aunts sitting in our home visiting us here in Maryland in February were now gone. I lost myself in deep grief, anxiety, and loss.

Professionally, I had this great perspective because I had all this knowledge, all this information, all this insight about pandemics. I knew how serious they were and how serious they can be—how they fundamentally changed societies politically, economically, socially, and technologically. And it was now unfolding before my eyes. I also felt an incredible, deep frustration with many individuals. The disappointment came from the fact that our society wasn't coming together to help address this pandemic.

Then it became even worse—civil unrest, strife, and conflict. My frustration grew deeper, along with my disappointment.

However, I emerged from this disappointment, frustration, and grief. I remembered the words I had written in my book, *The Art of Human Care*. They were exactly what I needed. Now I feel more passionately than ever that having a purpose and personalizing my care will help me adapt and evolve from this experience, one that everyone is going through. I personalized the issues for myself because I was going through a very personal kind of loss. During this time of COVID-19, I also decided that I wanted to help people find their purpose again. Because I had done that for myself, I was able to emerge from the funk and evolve through this terrible pandemic we all were dealing with.

However, most importantly, during COVID-19, I concluded that partnerships were what I needed to alleviate the frustrations I was having. Instead of arguing, fighting, worrying, and thinking if we should do this or that, we needed to rally together.

When I am involved in an organ transplant case, one person does not make a single decision about who will get a transplant. A panel that includes physicians, surgeons, social workers, nurses, psychologists, behavioral health professionals, and others first assesses the patient. Then they make a decision collectively. They ask, "Is this the best therapy for this individual? Is this the best course of action for them?" An entire team of people comes together in partnership to make it all happen.

We Need to Make the Most of It

We are all going to die. So whatever happens along the way, you know you can temporize and ease some pain and suffering. You can try to give the ill and suffering a little more life and a bit better life. But at the end of the day, we're all going to pass away. We have limited time here on earth—we need to make the most of it. You don't have to be a physician to heal. Giving someone inspiration helps heal them.

I've had patients who were terminally ill. I could not do anything medically for them. There was no medicine, no surgery, no way I could cure them. But I still find a way to partner with them in their care. You don't have to cure in order to heal.

Healing is deeply human, and you don't have to be a doctor with a medical degree to do it. You have to be a human being who cares about another human being—one human being willing to give another what they need at the time to lift their soul and lift their spirit.

Think about where you are in life. Think about the fact that you're alive today when so many people are not. In our country alone, we lost more than 400,000 people by mid-January 2021 to COVID-19. That's in our country alone. Those people are not here with us anymore.

COVID-19 placed all of us in an existential crisis—ourselves, our families, the leaders of organizations, and the leaders of our country. We all need to take time to look at the existential threats in front of us and figure out how to evolve—how to thrive. We can lean on partnerships to help. Amazing things can be accomplished by building a coalition, whether that coalition consists of colleagues, friends, or family.

If you are reading this book, I am partnering with you. Think about what you have to be grateful for, and start every day with that. You'll make every day a new day and every day a better day.

There's a magic happening. And you can be part of it.

Partnerships and Possibilities: Rolling Out the Vaccine

"This will be the most consequential professional achievement of your career," admonished my friend and colleague. In 2016, I passed the certification exam for the Subspecialty of Clinical Informatics. Just a few years before, 2016, I asked someone what clinical informatics is. The answer was not entirely clear then, and many have since made attempts to define it more simply. The American Medical Informatics Association (AMIA) defines clinical informatics as "the application of informatics and information technology to deliver healthcare services." According to the Healthcare Information and Management Systems Society (HIMSS), clinical informatics "promotes the understanding, integration, and application of information technology in healthcare settings." The Accreditation Council for Graduate

Medical Education (ACGME) defines clinical informatics as "the subspecialty of all medical specialties that transforms health care by analyzing, designing, implementing, and evaluating information and communication systems to improve patient care, enhance access to care, advance individual and population health outcomes, and strengthen the clinician-patient relationship." Wow! Indeed, the lessons of Professor Porter for simple elegance and genius are needed. I was intrigued by the information and technology references in my quest to understand this burgeoning 21st century clinical discipline better. In my work of thoracic surgery, my entire career was influenced by the use of information and technology to improve my patients' outcomes. Just decades ago, it was impossible to stop a patient's heart and perform surgery without the patient dying. Now, such procedures are done routinely every day around the world. Technology and information made the impossible possible.

Thus, I had an immediate interest in a clinical subspecialty that advanced technology and information. My simple definition for clinical informatics became the "use of information and technology to help others do their work better." Later I would read Charles P. Friedman's perspective and his description of clinical informatics as "the relentless pursuit of making people better at what they do." I was hooked. I immediately recognized the transformative potential for this discipline to impact healthcare, and I wanted to become an expert in every aspect of clinical informatics. Outstanding mentorship, excellent experiences working on challenging problems, and opportunity culminated in my appointment as the Chief Medical Informatics Officer (CMIO) for the United States

Navy. My colleague was right. Clinical informatics was very consequential and created many possibilities.

*In the fall of 2019, a cosmic chain of events occurred. The scheduled keynote speaker for the Annual American Medical Informatics Association (AMIA) Conference was canceled. By chance, I was consequently invited (as a remote backup to the original headliner) to be the opening keynote speaker at the Fall 2019 AMIA Conference in Washington, DC. The invitation came at a time of transition for me. I served as the Navy's Chief Medical Informatics Officer (CMIO), learned much, and was embarking on advancing many artificial intelligence initiatives to use information and technology to help others do their work better. I was relentless in my commitment to make people better at what they did. I prepared exhaustively for my presentation and delivered a keynote called "The New Dawn of AI, Health, and Creativity." My presentation centered on the human care themes of **purpose, personalization,** and **partnerships.** The message was well-received. After my keynote, many conference attendees and colleagues asked about my work at the Department of Defense. Specifically, people wanted to know how to apply data analytics, AI, and modeling to address clinical problems. They also wanted to know how they could use and leverage AI at their institutions and organizations to address clinical challenges. The questions engendered a desire for me to make our work more practical and espouse the power of partnership and possibilities.*

As the COVID-19 pandemic gripped the nation in the spring of 2020, our team in the Department of Defense rapidly assembled to analyze COVID-19 related data and support the nation's response to the pandemic under a project called Salus, named for the Roman goddess of safety and well-being. We established a team to build, develop, deploy, and scale the Salus platform. We rapidly analyzed data, planned, iterated, deployed, and scaled the platform to help inform prioritization of resources and guide decisions for individuals leading the COVID-19 response. We developed a multi-factor risk model for severe COVID-19 disease and reported the combined clinical and socioeconomic risk factors for COVID-19 related hospitalizations and deaths for populations. Eventually, using information and technology, we could predict individual probabilities of COVID-19 hospitalization for people, perform risk stratification, and map population risk levels at the county and zip code levels on a nationwide dashboard. Collectively, our partnership would help inform public health officials, plan vaccine prioritization, and assist leaders in the pandemic response. We applied the principles of purpose, personalization, and partnership and leveraged information and technology to help others do their work better.

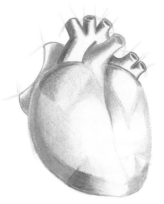

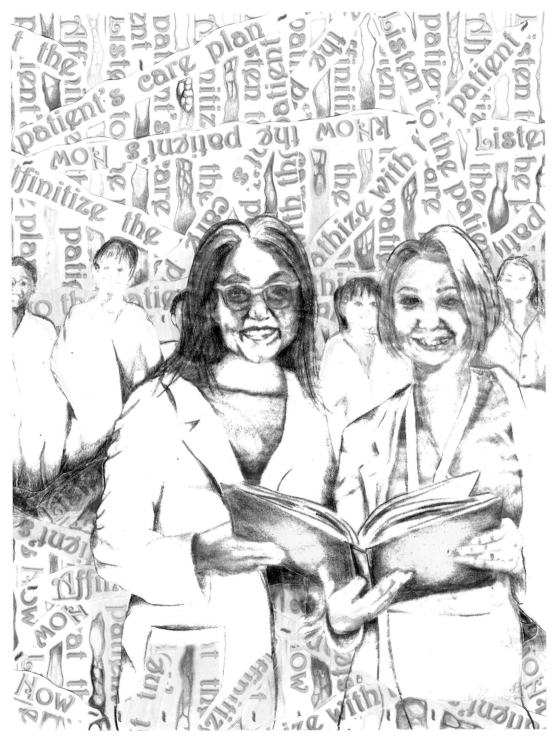

L.E.A.R.N. LISTEN. EMPATHIZE. AFFINITIZE. REPEAT. NOW.: Understanding Sowerby

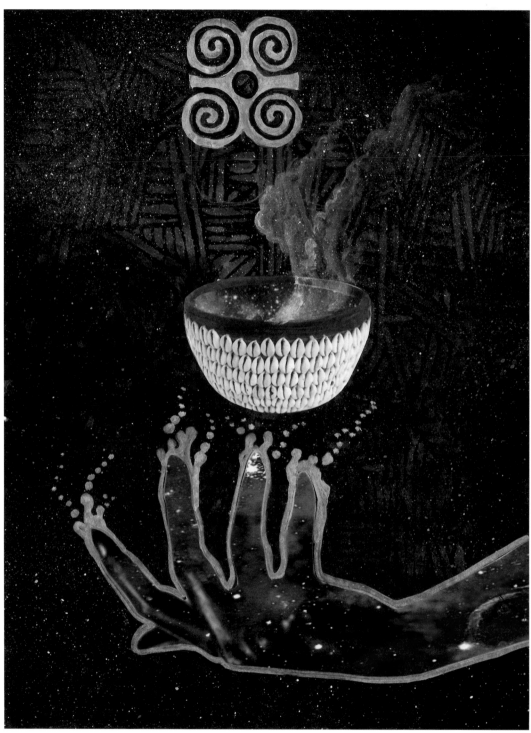

SOUP FOR THE SOUL: Massah Fofana

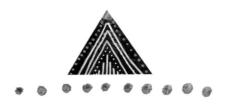

Chapter 9

Chicken Soup
for the COVID Soul

Jack Canfield, author of the best-selling *Chicken Soup for the Soul* series, has become my coach and mentor. I've learned a tremendous amount of wisdom from him. Plus, he possesses the rare combination of simultaneously being humble, a genuinely nice guy, and a brilliant person. Jack interviewed me shortly after my book *The Art of Human Care* was published. Here's just a little bit of that interview I want to share with you, for it is a prescription for what is needed most now. While my answers relate to those working in the realm of medical care, they can more broadly apply to any among you who seek a life with purpose, understand the importance of creating strong personal connections on and off the job, and appreciate the role partnerships play in creating success. As my preceding chapters have attempted to establish, the tenets of purpose, personalization, and partnership are the essential framework needed to evolve our world out of the pandemic and into a healthier future.

Dr. Tetteh: When I was an undergrad and junior, I was diagnosed with bacterial meningitis. I almost died.

Jack Canfield: I hear that not too many people survive that.

Dr. Tetteh: Yes. I had just been interviewed at medical school, Johns Hopkins, and I was on cloud nine. I came back to my small arts and science college in upstate New York. I became very ill, and about a week later, I was in the hospital. Thanks to the great doctors there, they figured out what was going wrong.

I had a tube in every orifice in my body and knew and understood profoundly what it meant to be a patient. And that experience, I think, has guided me in terms of how I approach healthcare. I ultimately didn't get accepted to Johns Hopkins, but that thought of knowing that I was going to be a physician, I think, kept me going.

So, I try to find out what my patients want to live for. I know it is one of those things that's intangible. It's unlike medicine. It's the one thing that a person is holding on to. If they have a purpose, you can get them to rally around an illness, condition, or setback. I was so excited that I was going to become a doctor, and that kept me alive. It gave me this great purpose.

Human care to me embodies all the significant care elements that were rendered to me when I was a patient, and in turn, knowing how impactful that was and how they saved my life. I want to return that to others. And our healthcare system has many great things about it, but sometimes it's not necessarily delivering human care.

Jack Canfield: We'll talk about that for a moment. I mean, we all talk about healthcare, we want healthcare, and all the politicians are talking about healthcare and whether it should be free or not and all that. How does healthcare differ from human care?

Dr. Tetteh: Well, three elements have come to embody what I describe as human care—purpose, personalization, and partnerships.

Again, I talk about this purpose—understanding your purpose as a healer, as a provider, and trying to appreciate the purpose of the person you're taking care of. I'm personalizing their care. I've had patients who have had a spectrum of diseases. With each patient, their circumstances are different. Their physiology is different. Their social conditions are unique. You have to personalize the care you're going to deliver to someone—to understand if it will be practical and useful for that individual. It's providing the right care to the right person at the right time— personalizing.

Partnerships are the third principle of human care. I think those elements embody human care. Healthcare, to me, is more sick care. You're sick. We give you some pills. We send you on your way. That's not trying to figure out what all of those other determinants of your health are, not taking time to understand what drives you, what keeps you going. Indeed, we are not personalizing care. Do you have pneumonia? I'm going to give you this, and you go on your way. Do you have a sore foot? I'm going to provide you with that, and you go on your way. In this scenario, I'm certainly not partnering with you because I may never see you again. I think that's the difference. Human care has a lot more comprehensive flavor to it.

Jack Canfield: Why do you think most doctors aren't doing that?

Dr. Tetteh: Ah, there are a lot of reasons for that. I think a lot of us enter the profession with an altruistic kind of view. I know I certainly did. We want to save the world. We want to make a big difference. Many stressors and so many barriers prevent us from being able to do that on a day-to-day basis. You have to keep seeing patients. And it takes time to develop a relationship with the patient truly. However, it's not impossible. It can be done.

Jack Canfield: Let's talk about that. I mean, I think most doctors say, "Well, I've got a stream of people who want to see me." I know for most people, when they try to get in to see their doctor, sometimes it's three weeks or a month out before they can get into the office. How can a doctor find the time and provide more patient-centered care?

Dr. Tetteh: Well, that's a great question. I think it starts foundationally and presently with communication. Being in the military, I've learned that communication is a crucial thing. I had a marine colonel tell me one time, "You know, Marines do three things. We move, we shoot, and we communicate. And when we don't do the third thing right, a lot of things go wrong." The same is true in healthcare and life.

If you don't communicate very well with your patients, you may not understand what the issue really is. And to address the issue of having that time, that constraint, it doesn't take a lot of time to listen to a patient. Most patients—and we've done studies on this—are interrupted by their care provider within the first 16 to 18 seconds of an encounter. That means the nurse, the doctor, and the allied health professional who's seeing them when they're seeking help interrupt the patient well before they can communicate their problems.

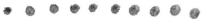

Jack Canfield: You mean the patient starts to talk, and the doctor interrupts them?

Dr. Tetteh: Correct, the patient is likely to be interrupted with a question or with a qualifier or something. If you think about being a patient—again, I remember what it was like to be a patient—in that gown, lying there, you're intimidated, scared, and nervous. And you're there, in your moment with the doctor, and you're afraid. They're telling you something, or they're about to talk to you, and they say, "Well, what brings you in today?"

Well, you begin to answer, and you are almost immediately interrupted with a question or comment. Now you've lost your train of thought. You're already scared. And you haven't been able to tell your story. By the end of the engagement, 10 or 15 minutes may have elapsed, and your time is up. The doctors may have asked you many other questions that may or may not be relevant to your particular situation at that moment in time.

You leave that encounter disappointed and unfulfilled, not having your issue, your problem, addressed. And the doctor potentially misunderstood or did not get a real sense of what you needed at that moment. The patient and the doctor have lost that moment. The doctor may have to reevaluate because that patient achieved no resolution during the visit or was sent back to a referring physician or someone else. And that is inefficient and wastes a whole lot of time. I tell my residents and my medical students, "Take the time to listen to a patient. Give them space. If you listen to the patient, they'll tell you the diagnosis if you truly listen to them. They'll tell you what's wrong with them."

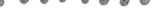

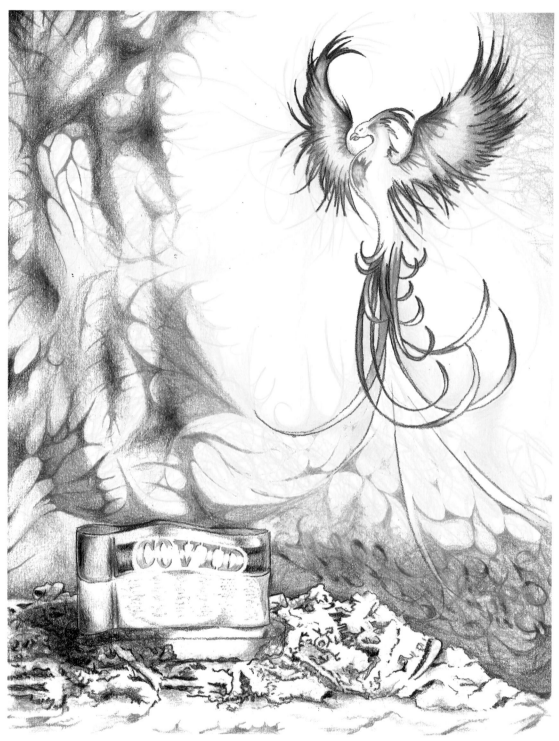

PHOENIX RISING: Understanding Sowerby

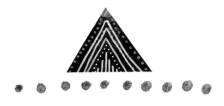

Afterword

Thomas Moran, PhD

Pandemics cause great suffering and kill human beings in terrifyingly large numbers. They also change the social and political landscape in utterly unpredictable ways. Perhaps among the most striking examples of such changes are the rise and fall of democracy in human history as closely tied to pandemics. Ancient Athens, the first prominent example of democratic governance, was so weakened by a pandemic that it couldn't survive its rival Sparta's attacks. Fifteen hundred years later, the Black Plague in Europe shook the foundations of the existing centralized authority and enabled democracy to emerge.

It is with these unique insights that Hassan Tetteh begins this quietly learned and wonderfully wise book. All of us living through COVID-19 are keenly aware of the dangerous threats it poses to our world and our own lives. Hassan enables us to see the possibilities for good in moments like this. Only someone with his background could write this book. He is a skilled heart-lung transplant surgeon and Naval officer, playing a pivotal role in harnessing Artificial Intelligence's capabilities to heal the wounded and promote health.

He has served as a combat trauma surgeon in Afghanistan, and he has broad training and experience in public policy formulation. But most of all, he is a deeply compassionate human being.

I have known Hassan for over 25 years since he was an undergraduate student leader in the college where I was the provost. We are both grateful to recognize that our relationship is like that of a father and a son. So I have long felt pride in his achievements. But when I read the first draft of this book, I was awed by what he had achieved. There is profound wisdom here; wisdom made clear, palpable, and accessible—an understanding around which a good life can be constructed by any of us no matter what our role.

Hassan's professional experiences are remarkable, and he seems to be superhuman. He is. But still, he is human. And the way he shares his fears and frustrations gives this book a particular resonance.

To know Hassan, even if only through his writing, is to see a person of unusual humility, dignity, and capacity to care about others. His profound love for his family and his unshakable decency are evident on every page of this book. What is also apparent both in Hassan's life and in the perspective he offers here is that character is not merely bestowed upon any of us; it is an achievement. And like any worthy achievement, it requires a determination to do something good and understand how we might do it. Hassan helps us see this, and in his formulation of "purpose, personalization, and partnership," he identifies bright stars to help us navigate through the dark night of this pandemic.

Hassan is not the first person to remind us that pandemics need not lead to endless despair and that instead, they can teach

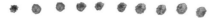

us how to live admirably, even hopefully. In the middle of the 20th century, Nobel Laureate Albert Camus wrote an influential novel called *The Plague.* It is a symbolic depiction of the way the members of a city respond to a devastating pandemic. Some citizens respond with cowardice, others with personal opportunism, many with indifference. But the central character, a doctor named Rieux, is the novel's commanding moral presence. He realizes they cannot let the afflicted suffer alone. He knows that their response to the pandemic defines their humanity. They must not yield to despair and abandon one another. He stolidly refuses to let the plague defeat the commitments of the community. But Rieux is world-weary. He hardly conveys a sense of bright hopefulness. Despite the suffering Hassan has seen as a physician and the horrors he has experienced as a combat surgeon, he retains an unbroken sense of hope.

I have recently read some psychological research that suggests that compassion and empathy, while similar, are not identical, and they affect different regions of the brain. Strong empathetic emotions are associated with areas of the brain related to depression. Strong, compassionate reactions are connected to happiness. This research is not conclusive, but it suggests that empathy opens us to others' pain, but compassion enables us to believe that we can alleviate pain. The former can lead to its own form of pain. The latter will galvanize us to action and pull us into a better future.

Hassan finds genuine joy in healing. The ideals of service are his North Star. He brings those qualities together in this inspiring book. It is transformative. No one can read it and think the same way again about contagious illness, healthcare, and our shared

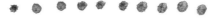

humanity. He shows us that pandemics have caused people to die, but if we look carefully and learn from what we see, they can also teach us how to live.

Thomas Moran, PhD
Director Emeritus, Institute for Ethics in Public Life
Distinguished Service Professor, Emeritus
The State University of New York at Plattsburgh
Plattsburgh, New York

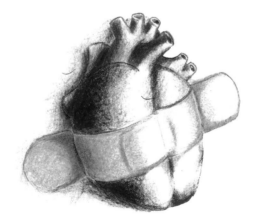

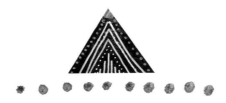

Acknowledgments

Hassan A. Tetteh

First, this book would not exist without the service, care, sacrifice, and compassion of all who have cared for another human. I am incredibly thankful to those who work every day in our places of healing to do the hard work of restoring health and wellness. These individuals deserve all the honor.

I am indebted to the many patients I met over the years, for they provided inspiration and wisdom. Stories and drama connect more effectively with people than facts and random words. Thus, Nikias and Hippocrates's story was adapted from a book called *The Sublime Engine: A Biography of the Human Heart* by brothers Stephen and Thomas Amidon. Professor Dorsey Armstrong's lecture on *The Black Death: The World's Most Devastating Plague* from *The Great Courses* provided invaluable context to characterize COVID-19 for the present day.

My teachers, mentors, and coaches have directly and indirectly influenced this work and taught me the healing art of medicine. The conceptual, editorial, and artistic works of Elijah Wells, Jill Block, Stoney Trent, Karen McDiarmid, Estelle Slootmaker, Alafaka 'Alee'

Opuiyo, Understanding Sowerby, Massah Fofana, Jack Canfield, Craig Poliner, Dr. Kevin Pho, and Greg Salciccioli were priceless.

Finally, the most thanks must go to my family, especially my wife Lisa, son Edmund, and daughter Ella for tolerating and supporting both a surgeon's and an author's schedule. Thank you all for always listening at the kitchen table to endless recitals, for enduring many drafts and revisions, and for your patience, love, and support with tea, a special treat, and warm embraces throughout many days and long nights. You are all a blessing. I am fortunate to have all of you, and I thank God for you every day.

Hic Pro Bonus
Here for Good...

Hassan A. Tetteh, MD
Poolesville, Maryland

References

Hippocrates (2012). *Aphorismi* (Latin edition). Ulan Press.

Amidon, S., & T. Amidon (2011). *The sublime engine: A biography of the human heart*. Rodale Books.

Armstrong, D. (2016). *The Black Death: The world's most devastating plague* (course guidebook). The Teaching Company.

Barry, J. M. (2018). *The great influenza: The story of the deadliest pandemic in history*. Penguin Books.

Frankl, V. E. (1992). *Man's search for meaning*. Rider Books.

Lynch, D. (2006). *Catching the big fish: Meditation, consciousness, and creativity*. TarcherPerigee.

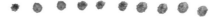

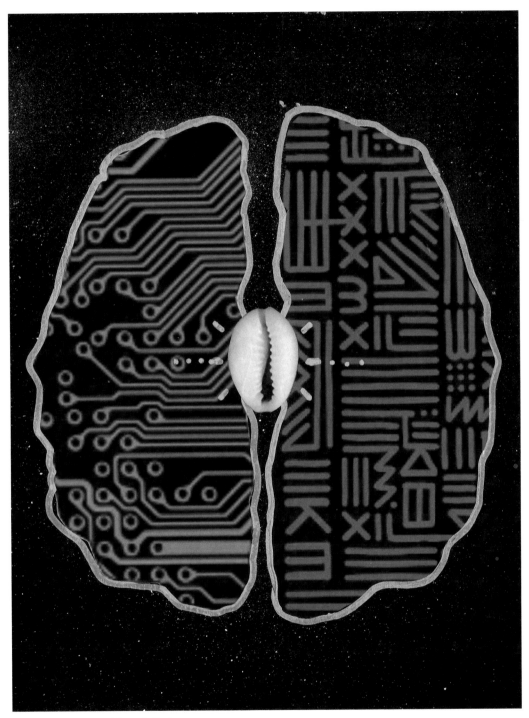

LISTEN AND LEARN: Massah Fofana

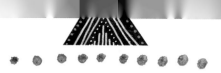

About the Author

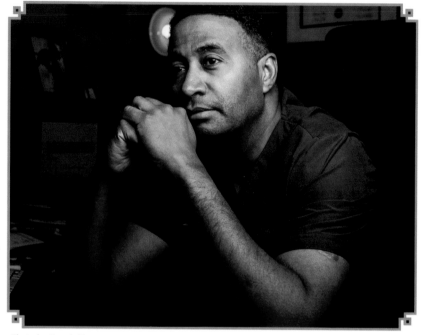

Photo by Angela Vasquez

DR. HASSAN A. TETTEH is a U.S. Navy Captain, an Associate Professor of Surgery at the Uniformed Services University of the Health Sciences, and adjunct faculty at Howard University College of Medicine. He was selected a 2019 Emerging Leader in Health and Medicine Scholar by the National Academy of Medicine. Currently, Tetteh is a Thoracic Surgeon for MedStar Health and Walter Reed National Military Medical Center. He leads a Specialized Thoracic Adapted Recovery (STAR) Team in

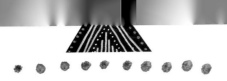

Washington, DC, and his research in thoracic transplantation aims to expand heart and lung recovery and save lives.

A native of Brooklyn, New York, Tetteh received his BS from State University of New York (SUNY) at Plattsburgh, his MD from SUNY Downstate Medical Center, his MPA from Harvard's Kennedy School of Government, an MBA from Johns Hopkins University Carey Business School, and an MS in National Security Strategy with a concentration in Artificial Intelligence from the National War College. He completed his thoracic surgery fellowship at the University of Minnesota and advanced cardiac surgery fellowship at Harvard Medical School's Brigham and Women's Hospital in Boston.

Tetteh is the founder and principal of Tetteh Consulting Group, creator of *The Art of Human Care* book series, and a best-selling author of several books, including *Gifts of the Heart, Star Patrol,* and *The Art of Human Care.* Tetteh is board certified in thoracic surgery, general surgery, clinical informatics, and healthcare management. He is a Fellow of the American College of Surgeons, a Fellow of the American College of Healthcare Executives, and a Fellow of the American Medical Informatics Association.

Tetteh received the Alley Sheridan Award from the Thoracic Surgery Foundation for Research and Education, was named a TEDMED Front Line Scholar, and is a TEDx speaker. He's an alumnus of the Harvard Medical School Writers' Workshop and the Yale Writers' Conference and lives near Washington, DC, with his wife, son, and daughter.

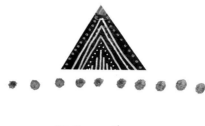

Kudos

"Dr. Tetteh is a shining example of the great people we have, and will always need, in the medical field. *The Art of Human Care for COVID-19* captures personal, powerful stories that will inform, inspire, and encourage us to keep the main thing the main thing no matter what crisis comes our way."

Dominique "Dom" Brightmon, Bestselling author and host of the *Going North* podcast

"As a transplant surgeon and combat Navy physician, Dr. Tetteh is intimately familiar with the gift of life and the end of life. He has written a poignant and compelling narrative that makes clear that the physician cannot be separated from his patient and community. As an African-American physician that hails from Brooklyn, that message is significant since too often education and achievement are used to separate clinicians of color from their own communities. Dr. Tetteh has weaved together a series of illustrative stories that show how our professions and our communities are intertwined. The humble *Art of Human Care for COVID-19* is a refreshing account of how clinicians can and should be advocates and empathetic and purposeful partners to their patients delivering tailored, personalized care. He carefully shows us the emotional side of the caring physician."

Ruth C. Browne, SD, President & CEO of Ronald McDonald House New York

"*The Art of Human Care for COVID-19* is authored by a humble and highly respected physician who genuinely cares about his fellow human beings, whether they are his patients or not. In his chapter about purpose, Dr. Tetteh states, 'Every day I'm reminded how precious life is.' That's the essence of both the author and this profound and inspirational book. Tetteh encourages the reader to value their life to the fullest extent possible and to embrace their ultimate purpose, particularly during this time of the COVID pandemic crisis. Read this book. You will definitely be better for it!"

Dick Bruso, Founder of *Heard Above the Noise*

"In his insatiable purpose to heal, Dr. Tetteh has found the words and the art to offer us an enlightening beacon of hope to overcome the darkness of COVID-19. A surgeon and military leader on the front line, also wounded by the loss of loved ones, Dr. Tetteh tells a fascinating tale of pandemics throughout history which enabled needed changes, empowering each of us to be part of the change the world needs today as we confront COVID-19."

Bettina Experton, MD, CEO Humetrix

"Beautifully and a timely written story by Dr. Hassan Tetteh, enhanced by his placement of the events of COVID-19 in historical perspective. His reaction to personal and professional loss urges and inspires us to find purpose in life during these challenging times, and should be a must-read for caretakers everywhere."

Gail Fraser-Farmer, MD, Internist at Long Island Select Healthcare

"Dr. Tetteh's book, *The Art of Human Care for COVID-19*, is refreshing, allowing us a glimpse into the mind of the author facing a pandemic as a transplant surgeon, as well as grieving personal loss as husband, father, nephew, and friend—a tragedy that now befalls so many other people here and elsewhere. COVID-19 has brought the entire world to its knees, some for days, some for months, willing us all to explore a renewed purpose within the confines of a disrupted life."

Tabitha Goring, MD, Associate Attending of Medicine at Memorial Sloan Kettering Cancer Center

"In *The Art of Human Care for COVID-19*, Dr. Hassan Tetteh not only opens your eyes to the long-term human effects of the 2020 pandemic, but also the history of how pandemics have changed human life over time, and some compelling thoughts on dealing with it personally."

Fred Katz, Senior Professional Faculty at Johns Hopkins University Carey Business School

"In this COVID-19 survival guide, Dr. Tetteh ushers you through a historic journey of how pandemics are likely the most powerful phenomenon in the restructuring of human civilization. *The Art of Human Care for COVID-19* requires a deep look inward. He will challenge you to do like Hippocrates and "burn it all down," everything you thought you knew pre-COVID, and reinvent a new purpose, a new you. A must-read for healthcare providers."

Edward Lathan, MD FAAEM, Emergency Physician

"At the core of *The Art of Human Care for COVID-19* is heart. Dr. Tetteh's writing is a leading edge, breath of fresh air, and inspires so much more than perspective around a pandemic. This book is both historically informative and deeply inspirational. It emphasizes the value of seeing the bigger picture of life and how we can allow COVID-19 to be a time of revolutionary renewal and rebirth within all of us. Dr. Tetteh provides light-bearing hope for all humans that elicits an internal knowing for the reader that we can and will move forward and be able to come out way better than ever imagined."

Kim O'Neill, Host of *Every Day Is a New Day* show/podcast and Transformational Confidence Coach

"Dr. Tetteh is a gifted surgeon, a trusted mentor and teacher, and an innovative and inspiring leader. In each of these roles, he is also as an artist— seeing problems and creating solutions in new and unexpected ways, always with a full and compassionate heart. In doing so, he touches all who are privileged to meet him in deep and meaningful ways. His latest book, *The Art of Human Care for COVID-19* provides a roadmap for all of us to have a positive impact on our world. I encourage everyone to read it. I find comfort and hope imagining what's possible if we all applied his Human Care Theory in our own lives."

Mary Sommer, Associate Director of Coaching and Education, Career Development Office at Johns Hopkins University Carey Business School

"From everyone who has been given much, much will be required; and from the one who has been entrusted with much, even more will be expected." Luke 12:48

"Dr. Hassan A. Tetteh's melding and amalgamation of historical perspective, personal experience, inclusive relevance, and most importantly, his human compassion, are a rare combination, and admirably conveyed with honesty and clarity in *The Art of Human Care for COVID-19*. At a time when the people of the world individually and collectively need encouragement, hope, and a vision, this work is a gleaming light of inspiration and direction for both the caregiver and those receiving care. It is the powerful 'shot in the arm' that we all really need at this time! This book is another 'gift' from the heart of Dr. Tetteh."

Randy Trowbridge, MD, Medical Director at Team Rehab/TechXercise and Past President of Fairfield County Medical Association

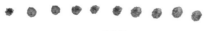

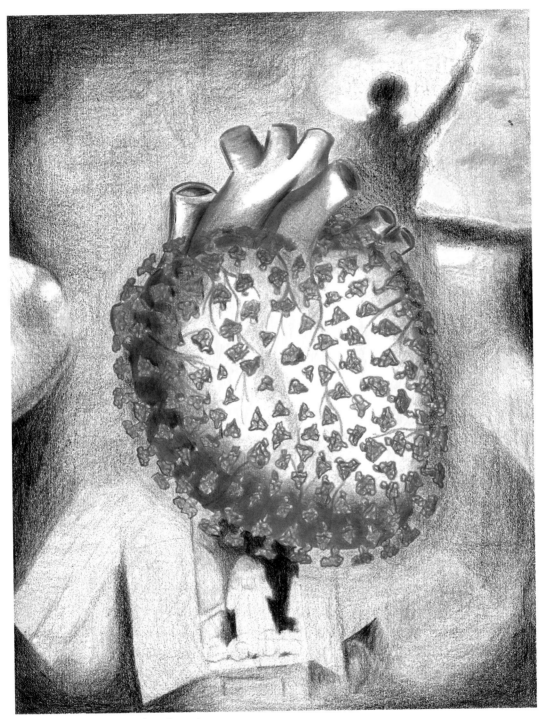

CIVIL UNREST: Understanding Sowerby

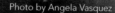
Photo by Angela Vasquez

"Art is not merely an escape from work,
but necessary to provide the energy and inspiration
to do the work even better. . . .
Art makes the work of healing better."

—Dr. Hassan A. Tetteh

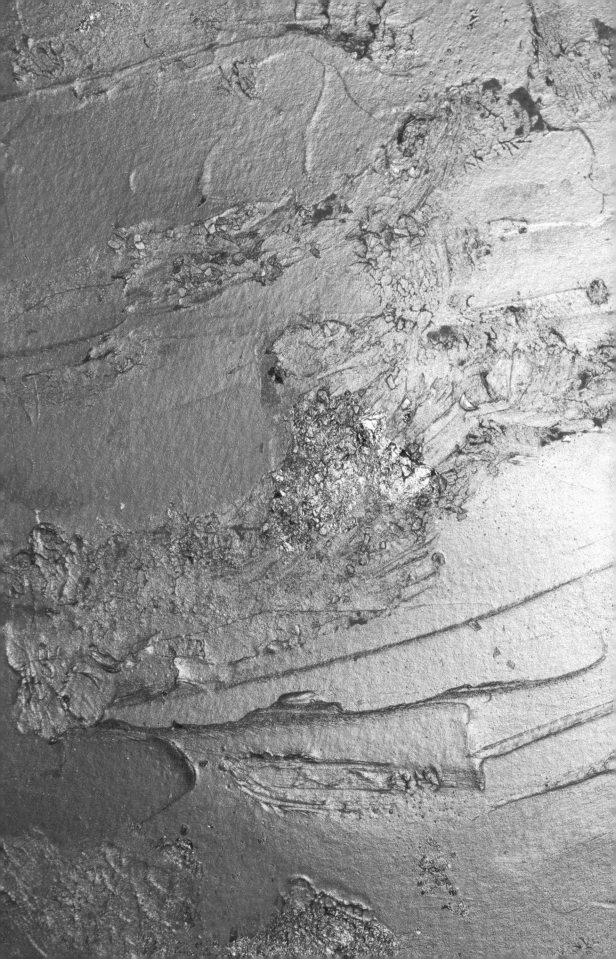